THE PRIME

THE PRIME

Prepare and Repair Your Body for
Spontaneous Weight Loss

KULREET CHAUDHARY, M.D.

INTEGRATIVE NEUROLOGIST

with Eve Adamson

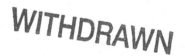

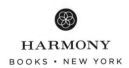

HARMONY

BOOKS • NEW YORK

Library of Congress Cataloging-in-Publication Data is available upon request.

ISBN 978-1-101-90431-2
eBook ISBN 978-1-101-90433-6

PRINTED IN THE UNITED STATES OF AMERICA

Book design by Elizabeth Rendfleisch
Jacket design by Christopher Brand

10 9 8 7 6 5 4 3 2 1

First Edition

Om Namo Narayani

CONTENTS

What you eat becomes your mind.
As is the food, so is your mind.

—Ayurvedic proverb

A NOTE TO READERS

The material in this book is for informational purposes only and is not intended as a substitute for the advice and care of your personal physician. As with all new diet and fitness regimens, this program should be followed only after first consulting with a doctor to make sure it is appropriate for your individual circumstances. Nutritional needs vary from person to person, depending on age, sex, health status, medication requirements, and total diet. *Specifically, this program should NOT be followed by women who are pregnant or breast-feeding.* The author and publisher expressly disclaim responsibility for any adverse effects that may result from the use or application of the information contained in this book.

PART ONE

Reverse Engineering
Our Eating

A NEUROLOGIST'S COMING OF AGE

My grandfather was a doctor for a large community of people in a town near Ludhiana in India. I loved and admired my grandfather, and I knew from an early age that I would be a doctor just like him. After an interview I did recently, I had a revelation: I am now practicing medicine much the way my grandfather did. But it wasn't always that way.

Life was much different in India in the 1970s than it is in the United States today. As the town doctor, my grandfather took his position as overseer of the community's health seriously. He created a partnership with the people of that community. When somebody got sick, he wasn't seeing the patient for the first time, in isolation, with no knowledge of his or her history or life. In most cases, he was also taking care of that sick person's parents, grandparents, and children. He understood how they lived. He created a loving bond with his community, and that bond allowed him to influence the entire family's health over the years. He didn't just provide a service. He provided a healing relationship.

When I was young, I was the apple of my grandfather's eye. I was the first grandchild and I was deeply attached to him. Up until I turned four, he watched me during the day and he took me into work with him regularly. I still have clear images of my grandfather in his little clinic caring for the people who came. There was always such a tremendous feeling of love and support there. He could be stern when he needed to be because he was invested in his patients' health, and they didn't always do what he told them to do. But it always came from love. Sometimes people could pay him and sometimes they couldn't, but that was never an issue. This shaped my perception of what medical care should be more than anything else I ever learned in medical school.

But then we moved to America. I was heartbroken to leave my grandfather, my extended family, and the community that nurtured me, but my parents were excited about the opportunities this new country would afford us. They wanted the American dream and they thought a better life awaited them. People in India envision America as shiny and exciting and full of opportunity, but I still remember the feeling of losing my foundation.

My parents, however, were eager to adapt. They moved my sister and me across the ocean and started a new life in Southern California. My mom was a physical therapist and my dad an electrical engineer. Although my parents discarded some of our customs (for example, our fully integrated Indian family, including my parents, grandparents, uncles, and aunts, was now split across two continents), we still practiced Ayurvedic medicine. This wasn't a big deal to us. It was just part of our lifestyle. Even though my grandfather had been trained in Western medicine, our culture practices a complete integration of "lifestyle medicine" with Western healing. If someone was sick enough to require medication, the doctor would prescribe it, but typically the first step was, "Hey, you have to change these things about how you are living." The goal was never to keep them on medicine, as it seems to be these days in the United States. Once here, we continued to live that way, including in the way we ate.

Of course we were introduced to some American foods we hadn't tried before, but our basic eating style remained rooted in Indian cooking. The spices we cooked with on a daily basis, which are now considered part of Ayurvedic medicine, were simply a part of everyday cooking, included turmeric, cumin, coriander, fennel, ginger, and amla berry pickle. It sometimes still strikes me as strange to "prescribe" to my patients what I used to know as pickles on the dinner table. I didn't know at the time that as we ate these foods, we were fighting diabetes, cancer, and obesity.

The way we dealt with minor health concerns was Ayurvedic in nature, too, although I didn't know to call it that at the time. For instance, if I got an ear infection, my parents would break out the garlic oil, which was just sesame oil with garlic cloves soaking in it. If any of us got bronchitis, my parents would give us a mixture of turmeric and honey. These were the first lines of defense, before ever considering antibiotics. I didn't get a lot of antibiotics growing up because our home remedies were so effective.

Another Ayurvedic concept we practiced was the portioning of our meals. Our lunches were really large, and dinners really small, and we always finished eating before sunset. It was simply a part of our culture and what we were used to doing.

I did notice some definite differences in the food between America and India. One of the most difficult was the milk. In India, the cows that are kept for milk production are treated kindly, like part of the family, and the milk tastes completely different. In India, milk tastes sweet. I used to love milk and butter in India, but I didn't like it so much here because it tasted bitter to me. It took me a long time to get used to it. I don't know if this is because of what the animals eat or how they are treated, but I do know that in India, the milk the cows give is voluntary (meaning they were not bred as dairy cows, to give us milk; we had milk only when they happened to have given birth). Also, the relationship between humans and animals is gentle and compassionate. I grew up feeling that and experiencing a gentle and natural relationship with food itself.

Yet we hardly ever had dessert. You might get some cake on your birthday, but other than that, fruit was the only dessert I knew. We craved fruit, and I remember how my father used to bring home boxfuls of mangoes. That was our dessert. I remember being seven or eight and we were allowed one sugary treat each week. It was always on a Friday and it was usually one of those miniature candy bars, like you get on Halloween. (Fridays were also when we were allowed thirty minutes of television—woo-hoo!) We enjoyed candy, but we didn't crave it because it seemed like such a rare event, and we didn't expect to be able to get it every day like kids so often do now.

I still don't have strong sugar cravings, and I suspect this is because I never developed a neuroadaptation to sugar. I'll talk more about this later, but when dopamine is released, triggered by sugar, the pleasure that results often gets mentally associated with the desire to be nurtured. When you experience it at a young age, this makes for particularly deep psychological as well as biochemical impressions. Both can become big challenges to overcome in adulthood. With this book, however, you have the tools to overcome them much more easily.

I also learned something when I was nine years old that is a fundamental part of Ayurvedic medicine: meditation. The loss of family support and community that we all experienced when we moved here took a toll on us. My mother went from raising two kids in a house with eight other adults to raising two kids essentially by herself. When she developed a thyroid condition called Hashimoto's thyroiditis, she went to see an endocrinologist, who told her the condition was related to the stress she was under. Even though he wasn't a meditator himself, he recommended Transcendental Meditation (TM) to her and she embraced it. Six months later, her thyroid condition was completely resolved and her thyroid function was perfectly normal. She figured that if meditation was able to normalize her thyroid, it could certainly do wonderful things for kids.

She sent us to a meditation teacher, someone I still remember with great fondness and whose presence always emanated such love, and my sister and I began to meditate, too. At this young age, I had found an extremely effective method for bouncing back from daily stress. (I'll talk more about this in the chapter on neuroadaptation, but stress has a huge influence on how well we process what we eat and how deeply neurochemical changes from food get rooted in our body. I believe that in addition to altering how I eat, my meditation practice has been the biggest contributor to who I am as a person today.) Because of meditation, I know how to go back to myself, no matter how stressful my environment. This is why I have such an appreciation for what meditation can do for the mind and body.

Yet despite my foundation, the American way of eating was bound to influence me, and perhaps it's no surprise that this happened when I was a teenager. I remember the first time I ever tried a corn dog. I was thirteen. Afterward, I got a horrible stomachache, nausea, and the strange sensation of feeling mentally cloudy. Yet after that, I began to eat processed food on a regular basis, simply because that was what my friends were doing. I didn't consciously connect my stomach issues with the food because, well, I was a teenager! All my friends were eating at fast-food restaurants on our way home from school, and of course I wanted to do what they did, to fit in. I now see that it was not a coincidence that I began to get sick more often.

Throughout high school, I began to experience bloating and tiredness after eating. Then, in college, I was diagnosed with irritable bowel syndrome (IBS) and prescribed Prozac because they said it was probably just stress. I knew it wasn't stress and I knew I wasn't depressed, so I never filled the prescription. The doctor never mentioned my eating habits. I gained ten pounds in college, and even though I still was slim, for me it was a sudden and uncomfortable change that coincided with my nonstop diet of traditional college food.

Then I began my medical training, and the situation only got worse. This was when I really began to lose my grip on the foundation of health my parents had provided. This happened because of a combination of several factors that anyone who has attended medical school knows all too well. First, I spent long hours studying and working. It was hard to find time to take care of myself. I didn't have time to cook, let alone sleep. I was happy when I got the chance to bathe every now and then! I still meditated, but even this became irregular. Second, even though I came into medicine with all this ancient wisdom, especially the belief that what you eat and how you digest it is directly related to why you get sick, everything I learned in medical school dismissed that notion. I learned there that you don't get sick because of digestion. You get sick because microorganisms enter your system. At first, I often asked questions and offered what I had grown up knowing, but time and again, everything I said was thrown out or criticized as archaic or backward. Little by little, I let go of the ancient wisdom in favor of what I thought was a superior understanding of the human body and how it works.

At age twenty, I still weighed just 115 pounds—pretty skinny for someone who is five feet, eight inches tall—but I didn't feel good. Then, slowly, so that I barely noticed, weight began to creep onto my skinny frame. I do remember feeling physically heavier and having less energy and clarity. I had always been good at putting complicated thoughts together, and I began to notice that I wasn't able to do that as well anymore. Every time I ate, I got sleepy. If you had asked me if my digestion was off, I would have said no, it's perfectly fine. Little did I know that I was wrong. It wasn't until I started having severe migraine headaches that I knew something was going in the wrong direction.

Finally, I graduated from my neurology residency and started my own medical practice, but life didn't get any easier. I took over the practice of another doctor, rather than coming into a doctor's office as an employee, as is more common. So right from the beginning, I was working fifteen-hour days. My health became something to put even further on the back burner. I just didn't have the time to focus on it, so I tried to ignore the headaches. They kept getting worse, however, and the excess weight kept creeping on. I wasn't paying any attention to the weight then, but the headaches were debilitating. I had to start my first prescription medication. Other than rare antibiotic use as a child, I had never been on anything other than home remedies and the occasional over-the-counter medicine.

This was illuminating. There I was, a neurologist, familiar with all the prescription medications out there, without ever having any direct experience using them. And they were absolutely horrible! I couldn't believe it. The side effects were so bad that I could barely tolerate them. This was what I'd been telling my patients to take? It was the first time I realized how miserable I was making them feel. I studied the list of side effects: weight gain, facial hair, memory problems, tremors, nausea, diarrhea, and so on. The first two alone disturbed me: weight gain and facial hair! If a medication makes you gain weight, that's a bad sign because it means the medicine is increasing your toxicity. One of the ways that your body deals with increasing toxins is to hide/segregate them into fat cells to protect your other organs from them. I began to notice that I could squeeze into my pants, but it wasn't comfortable. I switched to the only migraine medication that doesn't make you gain weight. It was called Topamax. It had been nicknamed "Dope-amax" by my patients, and I finally understood why. When I was on it, I could not think clearly. I had always been at the top of my class and now I was making to-do lists because I couldn't remember the most basic things. I had patients with complicated issues coming in to see me, and I was having to ask them to repeat things. This was not acceptable. It was the first time in my life that I felt stupid.

I began to get nervous, scared. I was in my early thirties, which is pretty young to be complaining about memory problems. Yet now I understood why my patients, some of them in their thirties, were complaining about the same thing—an inability to focus or remember things, even dementia symptoms. The medication I took to stop the headaches also gave me terrible neck pain. So there I was, stuck. I felt like I had two choices: I could suffer with debilitating headaches, or I could suffer from debilitating neck pain and give up my naturally sharp mind. I didn't know which was worse, but I suspected the headaches were the lesser of two evils. I used to look at my patients and think (or even say), "Suck it up. You have a medical problem. You need to be on medication." But when you become the patient, when you are on the other end of the stethoscope, and you aren't certain whether your medical problem or your medications are worse, only then do you realize there is something wrong with the way we are practicing medicine.

Finally, I told my mother about my situation. I told her I had terrible headaches but I couldn't tolerate the medication. I was so tired and groggy that I couldn't even run my practice. I asked her what I should do.

She certainly had an opinion. There was a group of Ayurvedic physicians who used to travel back and forth from India to the United States, and she connected me with one of them. She had taken me to Ayurvedic physicians a few times when I was younger (in fact, I was the youngest person in America at the time to have panchakarma, a traditional Ayurvedic health treatment). They had prescribed occasional small remedies, but it was never a big part of my life because I was never sick. This was the first time I ever went to see one of them with a real problem. So I went to meet one. The doctor was wearing a dhoti. This is the traditional dress for South Indian men, consisting of a long flowing white piece of cloth with gold and orange trim that is wrapped around the bottom half of the body like a skirt. I remember thinking, "Oh boy, here we go." After medical school, it just looked weird to me. It was all I could do not to roll my eyes. Despite being Indian, and despite my upbringing, my medical training had given me serious reservations and a certain degree of cynicism about this way of practicing medicine. If I hadn't been so miserable, desperate, and unable to tolerate my medication, I wouldn't have done it.

The first thing he did was sit me down and ask me about my digestion. This struck me as odd. I had headaches. He didn't even ask me about my headaches. My first response was that this guy had no idea what he was doing. I didn't have any digestive problems, so he was obviously focusing on the wrong thing. Next, he did a quick Ayurvedic physical. He looked at my tongue and my nails and he took my pulse. Then he gave me the verdict in a thick South Indian accent:

"You are very sick."

"No, I'm not," I said. "I just have headaches." I thought maybe he needed the reminder.

"No," he said. "Your digestion is very poor, and this is where all health problems begin. The headaches may be what you notice, but you are on your way to multiple health problems."

He was talking about my potential for disease, and he was talking to me as if I already had multiple diseases. To him, it was all connected because I was showing the first stages of the disease process. And that first stage is a disruption in digestion. Always.

"Do you get bloated?" he said.

"Yes," I said. "But everyone else around me does, too. Big deal."

"Do you get tired after you eat?"

"Yes, but doesn't everyone?"

Finally we talked about the headaches for a few minutes. He told me that he was certain I had a parasite infection. This surprised me. Not only had I never even considered that my headaches could be related to my digestion, but I certainly hadn't considered that parasites could be a cause. Sure enough, I was later diagnosed with giardia, which I probably contracted when I went to Africa at age nineteen. It had been a low-grade infection that had gone undiagnosed for years. Not only was this contributing to my ill health, the Ayurvedic doctor told me, but my poor habits developed during medical training and the loss of the good ones from childhood were also degrading my health.

His prescription was to start me on a few simple herbs. One of them was triphala, which had one of the ingredients that I remembered as a pickled berry from my childhood. He also gave me some basic dietary recommendations. I figured that his prescriptions would be easy to follow, and what did I have to lose?

Within three months, my migraine headaches were gone.

A BRIEF HISTORY OF AYURVEDA

Ayurveda, pronounced *I-your-vay-da*, means "knowledge of life," or "science of life," and it is the most ancient system of healthcare in the world. We don't know the exact origins of Ayurveda, but the legend is that it was handed down from Brahma (God) to humans through a lineage of sages in ancient India, who continued to develop and refine the practices through insight derived via deep meditation over five thousand years ago. These sages were not only holy men but also physicians, and Ayurveda was a complete system for managing all aspects of health as well as spirituality, including methods for increasing longevity, healing disease, performing surgery, cleansing the body, and addressing ethical dilemmas and spiritual development.

At first, Ayurvedic practices were handed down via an oral tradition, but eventually, they were written down, first in the Vedas, which are the four primary original spiritual texts of Hinduism (and one of the world's oldest religious texts, probably written between 1500 and 1000 BCE). At first, Ayurvedic medicine and Ayurvedic surgery were practiced separately, but eventually the system unified into one, as exemplified in three main Ayurvedic texts: the *Charak Samhita*, the *Sushrut Samhita*, and the *Ashtanga Hridaya Samhita*, all likely over 1,200 years old. They cover physiology, anatomy, disease and its causes and symptoms, diagnosis, treatment (including herbal and surgical), prescriptions, prevention, and longevity. Sub-branches include internal medicine; ear, nose, and throat medicine; toxicology; pediatrics; surgery; psychiatry; sexual and fertility treatment; and rejuvenation. It is an astoundingly complete system.

So what are we to make of it today? Did Ayurveda come from some divine source? Obviously, we can't prove such an assertion one way or the other, but don't be fooled into thinking there is no scientific basis for Ayurveda. On the contrary, what the ancient sages knew has been slowly proven throughout the ages, as science continues to catch up to this complete and life-transforming system of health maintenance, disease prevention, and cure. Ayurveda continues to evolve without ever abandoning its original construction. In fact, an important part of Ayurveda is not to reject any aspect of medicine that could help the patient, so it does not preclude the use of modern Western medicine. This is why it works so well for me in my practice—it is in line with everything I do, even when I am using aspects of my conventional medical education to treat my patients.

In other words, Ayurveda remains relevant and I see its profound effects every day with my patients as well as in myself and my family. I love it because it loops in all aspects of the self—the physical, the emotional, the mental, the spiritual—to treat the whole person in ways that modern science is now confirming are effective and based on scientific truth.

I was shocked. I had never had one single day of medical training that even suggested that neurological issues could be linked to the gut. I had seen multiple doctors and tried everything they suggested without any relief, and the solution had turned out to be so simple: just fix the gut. I wasn't just a little better. I was *headache-free and side effect–free.*

But it didn't stop there. Within the next six to nine months, my mental clarity got so good that the job that had been taking me fifteen hours—seeing patients and trying to improve the way the office was functioning—became easy and began to take much less time. I was ending my day sooner because the solutions to the problems I encountered every day were becoming obvious to me. My mind sped up again. I felt sharp and clear. My energy returned. Before, I never made plans with friends after 7 p.m. because I never knew if I would crash by then, but no more. I was finally starting to feel like myself—like the version of me I hadn't experienced since before medical school. It was exciting.

My physician colleagues all know that after you finish a medical residency, you feel like you have sacrificed some of your health and youth. We all learned that the only way to get a modicum of energy was to medicate with caffeine and stimulants. It's practically the first thing you learn in medical school! And yet there I was, getting my youth back. It was eye-opening to think that simple changes to improve my digestion were all that was required to reverse the clock. Even my skin looked better. It had more elasticity, and the wrinkles I was developing began to disappear. What I thought I had given up to my medical training was coming back to me!

The next thing I noticed was that the excess weight I had accumulated was falling away. I was getting smaller and less puffy. My clothes began to fit better. For the first time, I realized I had gone up a few clothing sizes. I had been so busy trying to be a doctor and managing my headaches that I hadn't realized I had gained an additional ten pounds during my neurology residency. Without me even trying, those extra ten pounds disappeared as my digestion got better.

That was when I hit a crisis in my professional life.

The way I was practicing medicine began to feel wrong. There I was, prescribing medications I myself wouldn't take. It felt not just medically wrong, but wrong on a human level. I knew I wasn't taking responsibility for my patients. I was bandaging their symptoms but I wasn't fixing them. I wasn't healing them. It was impossible not to think about my grandfather. What would he be doing in my position?

My colleagues already thought my visits to the Ayurvedic physician were a little weird. They warned me not to sacrifice my promising career. I could be a pioneer in neurology! I was being groomed for neurological greatness! And yet I was now realizing that I didn't want to be a pioneer in neurology. I just wanted to be a normal neurologist who helped people. And now, when my patients came to see me with neurological problems, I couldn't help but wonder: is this a gut problem?

This was, of course, total heresy.

Something neurologists have traditionally been taught is that the blood-brain barrier keeps the brain isolated from the rest of the body. The brain is supposedly immune to biochemical issues the lower body might experience. And yet I had seen and felt it firsthand: gut health is indeed tied to the nervous system. Today, scientists are finally discovering the reality of this, as we increasingly understand the brain-gut connection, the effects of gut bacteria on the nervous system (including that they manufacture most of the body's serotonin), and the complex network of neurons located in the gastrointestinal tract that has led many to dub the gut "the second brain." At the time of my professional crisis, however, this was not an accepted idea.

Nevertheless, when the Ayurvedic doctors I had visited came from India, I started taking some of my sickest patients to see them. These were the patients with multiple sclerosis (MS) and Parkinson's disease. I would sit in on their consultations to see how they would assess my patients. I didn't know how to become an Ayurvedic practitioner myself at that time, but I was curious what they would say. Of course, the doctors always began with questions about the digestion and the gut, and improving the digestion was always the first prescription. I watched my patients with MS having fewer relapses and getting off all the medications they were taking for the multitude of symptoms associated with the disease, as well as the medications to counteract the side effects of the other medications. They were getting off the medications for fatigue, constipation, depression, and urinary problems. My patients with Parkinson's were able to reduce their medication doses as well. Patients who had been having trouble walking were now taking dance classes. Many of my patients with Parkinson's even began to smile again, which is a function that is lost over the course of the disease as their faces become "masked."

At some point, however, as I began to take more and more patients to see these doctors, it became difficult to coordinate. I wanted all my patients to benefit from this knowledge, but there just wasn't time or availability. That was when I realized I had to get trained. I contacted a group that was doing a lot of research on lifestyle medicine, funded by the National Institutes of Health (NIH). I knew they used to train Ayurvedic physicians but hadn't done so in fifteen years. I told them I needed to be trained. They told me they were too busy doing research. I argued with them. I told them that I needed physicians to train me. It would be better than being trained by someone from India because they understood Western medicine, too. If they trained me, I could become a bridge between Ayurveda and Western medicine. I could connect the dots.

After a tremendous amount of convincing—I think they just got tired of me hounding them—they agreed to set up a course to train already-established physicians in San Diego in Ayurvedic medicine. Four doctors signed up, including me. By the end of the course, I went back to my practice convinced that I would have a hard time getting my patients excited about my new focus. I was wrong. It was exactly the opposite. Within four months, almost my entire practice consisted of an integrative approach of traditional neurology and Ayurvedic medicine. Patients were hungry for it. They weren't the obstacle to this new way of practicing. I had been the obstacle. I was the one with the hang-ups about how people would accept it. I discovered that many of my patients were already trying alternative treatments and strategies on their own but had been nervous about telling me. They were relieved to have a physician who was truly willing to partner with them in their health efforts.

My practice changed. I began each visit with a detailed three-page questionnaire for every patient. I looked at my patients differently, not just at their symptoms but at their lives. Little by little, as I transformed my practice, I began to see other members of my patients' families. In many ways I became not just a neurologist and an Ayurvedic practitioner but also a family doctor.

It was right around this time that I was the target of an intervention. A group of physicians I worked with took me out to dinner, and then they started in: "We think you are throwing your career down the toilet." "You are a young, bright neurologist and you are practicing voodoo." "Just look at this from a financial model. Even if you make your patients better, you will practice yourself right into bankruptcy because you won't have any patients left."

I remember trying not to freak out right there in the restaurant. Were they really suggesting that I shouldn't be healing my patients? But I was also laughing inside. I was getting an intervention for being a doctor who was making people healthy! That was when I realized, in a way I hadn't before, how far astray modern medicine has really gone. First, helping people change health-destroying habits is considered irrelevant to the practice of medicine. Second, healing people isn't good for business. These were good, well-meaning physicians; this was just what the culture of medicine had become. Needless to say, I did not heed their advice.

I am so grateful that I developed those severe migraine headaches. If I hadn't experienced how hard it was to be a patient and tried medications that were unbearable, I might never have been inspired to do what I do today. I had a great start in life, but my story shows you how quickly someone—even a healthy person—can get off track. Health can be disrupted so easily by the habits of modern life.

And my medical training? Now I know which treatments are "backward." Medical school is a sort of brainwashing. You are deprived of sleep while being constantly pressured not to think like an individual. You are discouraged from asking why. You can't even ask why someone is sick. Medical school teaches how to describe the disease and abnormal biochemistry, and what pharmaceutical agents to use to correct that abnormal biochemistry, but to ask why someone got sick in the first place is considered a naïve and foolish question. Isn't that supposed to be our job as physicians? To ask why? To get to the bottom of the cause? At last, I saw that the reason we aren't supposed to ask why is that our professors and attending physicians simply don't know the answers. It's a lot easier to say "Don't ask" than "I don't know."

I did well in medical school. I graduated in the top percentage of graduates in the nation (according to the Alpha Omega Alpha Honor Medical Society—the Phi Beta Kappa of medical school), but part of me started to die in that process. I was no longer able to be inquisitive, no longer able to be creative, and for the first time in my life, I was no longer taking good care of myself. Everybody around me was less healthy when they graduated compared to when they started, so none of this felt unusual until I looked at it in retrospect. All my colleagues felt like they were aging faster, everybody was gaining weight, and nobody felt particularly well after they ate. This was life in medical training. This is life for many in our crazy-fast modern world.

And yet this is not living.

I took a different path, and I spent the next decade formulating a new way of practicing medicine. I came up with a program, initially for the purposes of neurological healing, that is not like traditional neurology, nor like traditional Ayurveda. It combines the best of both worlds. I began with protocols to detoxify the body and reduce inflammation in the whole system, before ever asking my patients to make a single dietary change. I did this because I saw how hard it is for people to change. I witnessed how my patients' biochemistry was dictating the way they ate, and even the way they thought. It was controlling their choices and the direction of their lives. Until I could free them from that biochemical prison, they wouldn't be free to make the right choices. As my patients got cleaner and clearer, they naturally started making the choices I would have asked them to make up front. They often tell me things like, "I don't know what happened to my sugar cravings!" or "I can't eat the huge portions I used to eat anymore," or "The junk food I used to love just isn't appetizing anymore. It's so weird!"

And they began to lose weight. At first I didn't pay much attention to the weight loss. I was so caught up in improving brain health, stopping the progression of any neurological or other disease present, that weight loss seemed inconsequential. Sure, it was great, and probably good for my patients, but it wasn't the point. I was more concerned about fighting potentially life-threatening disease processes. But it didn't take long for me to notice that time and time again, after a few weeks of treatment for a neurological condition, many of my overweight patients were casually mentioning to me, "Oh, by the way, I'm losing weight. Thanks!" In fact, almost every overweight patient told me that, yes, he or she had lost weight. They would confide, "Dr. Chaudhary, I have to thank you! I lost twenty pounds," or "I'm down thirty pounds now, and I wasn't even trying!"

It couldn't be a coincidence. This curious and spontaneous weight loss had to be related to my neurological detoxification regimen. I began to track weight loss in my patients in a more systematic way, and sure enough, of those who had weight to lose, some lost a little, and some lost a lot. A few lost a hundred pounds or even more, but the average weight loss was between twenty and thirty pounds over the course of a three-month treatment protocol. Many of my patients who had struggled with weight issues for decades found themselves at a weight any body mass index (BMI) calculator would deem "normal." In many cases, this was weight they had been unsuccessfully trying to lose for years.

Weight loss was never an expectation I had for my patients. I'm a neurologist, not a weight-loss doctor. I'm not interested in calories and I never asked a single patient to count them. It never dawned on me that the way I was treating my patients for their neurological symptoms could have anything to do with treating weight issues—until I saw it for myself. It was undeniable. I was seeing significant spontaneous reductions in excess body weight, along with improved cholesterol levels, blood pressure levels, blood sugar levels, and of course, neurological symptoms. My patients looked thinner, felt more energetic, had less pain, and said they were thinking more clearly and quickly. They experienced fewer symptoms, such as memory issues, brain fog, joint pain, and sleep problems, and looked (and *were*) healthier.

It wasn't until the producer of *The Dr. Oz Show* asked me whether I had an effective weight-loss method that I suddenly realized I did. My method was what I give to every patient, but not for that reason. It's a program to rid the body of toxicity and inflammation, but in the process, the brain clears and the weight comes off.

It's funny that ten years later, I'm seeing all of these things that I was criticized for by the medical community becoming mainstream, as clinical trials finally reveal the scientific basis for the things Ayurvedic physicians have been saying for five thousand years. Even the spices that I grew up with in my mother's Indian kitchen are showing promise for fighting medical issues, reducing inflammation, facilitating immunity, and reducing excess body fat. We are discovering the links between the brain and body. We are discovering the power of lifestyle changes. It's all finally coming full circle.

But I'm not going to say "I told you so" to my former colleagues. I'm just going to keep practicing my unique form of integrative medicine. Ayurvedic physicians know that implementing multiple interventions is always more powerful than doing one thing at a time, and this is how I've designed my program. Now traditional physicians are coming to me as patients or referring patients to me, and although they sometimes tell me they don't understand why what I do works, they admit that it does work. I've had neurosurgeons tell me, "I don't know what you're doing, but your patients recover from surgery so much faster than other patients."

I was never looking for the kind of recognition I received by being a regular guest on *The Dr. Oz Show*, or by being named as a top doctor in San Diego. And quite honestly, I don't need it. Except that it does provide me with a way to help more people. I now have patients in my California clinic coming from Texas, New York, Oklahoma, Massachusetts, Mexico, and even England, because they can't get what I do anywhere else. I can't accommodate the demand. So I hope this book will give a foundation to the many people I can't see personally. The program in this book is what I do with almost every single one of my patients. It is a powerful beginning for anyone who tries it.

It was my purposeful divergence from conventional medicine that brought me back to my roots and also brought me recognition beyond anything I could have imagined. I am often interviewed by physicians and journalists and asked the question "How can we change medicine?" I'm realizing how simple it would be—yet it's going to take time. Changing medicine is about changing perception. It's about caring for your little village in your medical practice, and looking at not a body part but a life. If every single doctor told every single patient to (1) purposefully reduce stress (this applies to doctors, too!), (2) drink more water and less soda, and (3) poop once a day, I think that alone would have a profound effect on the world. Becoming this kind of a doctor has made me a better human being. I'm kinder, more compassionate, wiser, and more loving. I think one of the greatest casualties of modern medicine is the loss of the healing heart of the physician. People don't even recognize that doctors have become a casualty of modern medicine. I'm no longer a casualty. I got the opportunity to find myself.

My journey was never esoteric or ethereal, and it never involved conversations with angels or anything bizarre or supernatural. It started with my gut, and that's about as simple as you can get. What I'm most grateful for is that I am finally taking responsibility for my patients, much the way my grandfather always did. And now that includes you.

My great grandfather lived to be 104, where he remained a part of the community for his entire life. Each day in Ludhiana during his lifetime was nurturing on such a deep level of the human experience. I try to replicate that in my life today, and in the way I practice medicine. I'm re-creating the village I lost. I'm finally home.

CHAPTER 1

YOU'RE DOING IT BACKWARD

You're doing it backward.

If you are like the majority of people who have tried to lose weight, you've done it (or tried to do it) by going on a diet, or exercising more, or both. That's what you're supposed to do if you want to lose weight, isn't it? It's what doctors tell you to do. It's what nutritionists tell you to do. It's what most diet books tell you to do.

If you've tried to lose weight this way, maybe it worked. Maybe it didn't. Maybe you lost some weight, but gained it back. No matter what happened, the one experience you probably have in common with most others who have tried is this: *it was extremely difficult.*

Losing weight is hard to do. Or, it's hard to do the way people tend to do it. Even diets that claim to be easy often feel incredibly strenuous in practice. Sometimes the promise of a new diet is enough to keep you going for a while. Maybe you are all fired up about your new plan at first and you are okay for a week or two, but eventually the novelty of it wears off, the routine gets tedious, and your body cries out against the deprivation and the exertion. Diets typically deprive you of things you want—and the more you tell yourself you can't have those things, the more you want them. Whether the diet tells you not to eat sugar or fat or bread or meat or dessert or something else, it's hard not to eat the things you want. And if it has you counting calories or fat grams or carb grams, you're not only not eating what you want, but you also have to focus on constantly quantifying your consumption of everything you don't really want to eat. It's also hard to eat less than you are used to eating. You want more food! And it's hard to exercise if you don't have the energy, aren't used to it, and don't enjoy it. Maybe you tried to exercise but it was just too unpleasant, too time-consuming, too exhausting or painful, maybe even injurious.

In most cases, the urge to eat the foods that you're told got you in trouble becomes too strong. The temptation to skip one day of exercise, and then another, becomes overwhelming. Before the unwitting dieter knows what is happening, it's back to old habits again. Not long after that, weight goes back up, energy goes back down, thinking gets fuzzier again.

Maybe you think you know the reason for this: You are weak. You lack willpower. You aren't motivated enough. You are genetically destined to be fat and lazy. No! I am here to tell you that none of these things are true. If you blame yourself for your failure to lose weight, you are pointing your finger in the wrong direction.

Nobody wants to drag around excess body weight. Nobody wishes for low energy. Nobody loves brain fog, and nobody hopes to have an increased risk of disease. Yet here you are, despite what you want for yourself. How did it happen? It's not because you are weak. Not because you are unmotivated. The reason is simple: it's because you didn't realize the power your initial, often casual lifestyle choices would have over your future ability to make better choices. You didn't realize what the foods you chose were doing to your brain.

There is a specific and scientific reason why diets and exercise plans feel so punitive and even impossible: you have been trapped. Despite your best intentions, you have been locked in a biochemical prison. You have inadvertently become addicted to the things that put you in that prison, and now they are your prison guards. They keep you chained and they keep you behaving according to their wishes, not yours.

There is only one way to fight biochemistry: with biochemistry.

This is one of the first and most important things I would like every single overweight person to understand: Being overweight is a biochemical issue, not a personality flaw. My patients have been chiding themselves and disliking themselves, often for years, even decades, because they think they are too "weak" to lose weight. Yet when I think of the patients who come in to my clinic, I can't help but be impressed with how they have handled other areas of their lives. Many of them are extremely bright, talented, organized, and ambitious. Some have degrees in law, business, and medicine. They hold down difficult jobs or have built successful businesses from the ground up. They have risen through the ranks in their chosen field. They work hard. They create things. They are multitasking wizards who are able to support entire families. They have succeeded at many challenging projects, and they are motivated and self-directed. So why has losing weight been so hard for these people? It's certainly not because they are lazy. They clearly don't lack willpower in other areas of their lives. What they do lack is just one simple thing: an understanding of how their biochemistry is stacked against them.

This is wonderful news. No matter how long you have been over-weight, if you have the right biochemical tools at your disposal, you can cure your weight problem. There is no mystery to it. It's science, pure and simple. You don't have to change your personality. You don't have to acquire superhuman personal discipline. You don't even have to force yourself to stop eating cookies.

All you have to do is start shifting your biochemistry, bit by bit, in a different direction.

Imagine that you want to become a lawyer. You wouldn't just wake up one day and decide that if you just have enough willpower, you can go out and start practicing law. No, you need the right education and you need to earn the right degree. You need to go to college and then you need to go to law school. You go out and collect the tools that you need so you are prepared and qualified. Only then will you be successful.

Weight loss is exactly the same. You have to have the right tools to do it. You can't just do it through willpower. Thinking that weight gain is a personal failure of willpower is like saying that you should be able to stop a bullet using your willpower. You can't. A bullet is a physical phenomenon, and so is your weight. You don't stop a bullet by thinking. You get out of the way. Food has essentially become your biochemical bullet, but with the right strategies, you can dodge that bullet . . . and still get to eat.

The Food Industry's Strategy

But what caused this biochemical prison? We are meant to eat food; we need it to survive. So how did this life-sustaining substance grow walls and become a cell? Unfortunately, much of the problem is rooted in the quality of the food we eat. This isn't an accident. The food industry already knows better than anyone how closely biochemistry is linked to food choices and overconsumption; it's in their best interest to know it. Combining savvy marketing techniques with extensive study of the "bliss point," or the point at which sugar, salt, and/or fat provide the most euphoric combination in a particular food, these manufacturers have created products that people, once they are hooked on them, simply can't resist. They keep eating them, and they keep buying more.

The statistics bear out the food industry's success. According to the U.S. Department of Agriculture (USDA), the average person eats 152.4 pounds of sugar and other sweeteners and 74.5 pounds of added fats and oils such as salad dressing, cooking oil, frying fat, and butter every year. In fact, we're consuming more of just about everything—19 percent more calories since 1983, 57 pounds more meat per person since the 1960s (and a third fewer eggs), more cheese (but less milk), and 66 percent more fat since the 1950s. We're eating more fruits and vegetables, which is a good thing—20 percent more since the 1970s—and eating 45 percent more grain since the 1970s, along with a 39 percent increase in sugars since the 1950s.[1] And guess how much of your dollar goes to actual farmers?

Just 19 cents, compared to 81 cents for labor, packaging, transportation, energy, profits, advertising, and more food industry expenses.

The bottom line is that our increasing consumption, especially of cheap addictive foods containing a lot of highly processed sugars and fats, is profitable for them, but not for us. A recent study in the *Journal of the American Medical Association*[2] links increased sugar consumption by Americans in the last decade to increased mortality due to cardiovascular disease. Other studies link increased sugar consumption with the obesity epidemic[3] and correlate skyrocketing sugar intake with skyrocketing obesity rates.[4] Still other studies have demonstrated the link between fast-food habits and weight gain (and other health issues, especially related to blood sugar and insulin).[5] And that's just the tip of the iceberg. I could quote studies all day showing you the links between the way our food is processed to become addictive and our weight and health issues.

The point is *not* that you are making bad choices because you like being overweight and unhealthy. The point is that your weight gain has everything to do with the purposeful manipulation of food ingredients to create products most people are not biochemically capable of resisting for long. The foods most easily and cheaply available to people living in the modern Western world have been purposefully engineered to keep you coming back for more. Food scientists working for food companies know exactly how to get you hooked. The food industry knows more than the consumer, and they use that knowledge to get you to buy and eat what they are selling, whether it is nourishing or likely to induce excessive weight gain. Certain foods, especially processed and restaurant foods, contain a virtually irresistible mix of flavors and ingredients that light up the same parts of your brain as addictive drugs. As you fall under the spell of these tasty foods, you will find yourself eating more and more.

These foods gain a foothold in your system as they change your biochemistry in ways that make you dependent on the good feelings you get from those chocolate bars or potato chips or cheeseburgers, or even those "healthy" veggie burgers on big fluffy buns with extra avocado and a side of French fries and a vegan cupcake for dessert. You are overdoing it, plain and simple—and you can't help it. It's that perfect combination you'll find in pizza, or macaroni and cheese, or even a giant chef's salad with creamy dressing. These foods, especially when they are highly processed and eaten in certain combinations, can increase the toxic load in your body, turn on inflammation, and alter your biochemistry in a way that makes it extremely difficult for you to make independent and conscious choices about what to eat next. Even as you try to diet, your body will keep crying out for more, more, more. More sugar! More fat! More salt! Pile it on! You only live once!

Just to be clear, there is nothing wrong with natural sugar, or natural fat, or even natural salt. Fruit has sugar along with fiber and nutrients. Avocadoes have healthy fat and nutrients. Himalayan salt is unprocessed salt with minerals. What I'm talking about is when refined sugar, fat, and salt are added to natural foods to create an overload beyond what those foods themselves contain. This has a specific effect on the brain, which I'll explain later in this book. For now, just know that when you get used to extremely sweet foods or foods made with refined sweeteners such as white sugar and high-fructose corn syrup, fruit doesn't taste interesting anymore. When you get used to extremely high-fat foods or foods that are deep-fried or cooked with highly refined fats, then you may find yourself considering deep-frying your avocado (that's a thing—I've seen it on a menu). When you get used to extremely salty snack foods, then wholesome natural foods with a little sea salt don't feed your craving anymore.

The problem is, these fake foods aren't giving you the kind of energy or nutrition you need in balance with the calories they deliver. They also give you things you don't want—along with their addictive doses of refined sugar, fat, and salt, they deliver deleterious doses of toxic substances, such as artificial preservatives and food colors, ingredients that cause inflammation in your system. That's when things start to go wrong. What you thought was a healthy frozen entrée or a fun snack food or a tasty drive-through lunch is encouraging harmful biological processes inside your body, when all you meant to do was nourish yourself with something easy and pleasant. Before you know it, you are hooked—addicted to extreme sweet, extreme fat, extreme salt, and nothing else will do. Real food bores you because it doesn't get you "high." It's no wonder you couldn't stick to that diet you were so excited about last month. And the month before that. Your body is primed in the wrong direction.

Most weight-loss regimens expect you to make drastic changes from inside a body that isn't prepared to make them. When your body is in a toxic inflammatory state, "Just eat less and exercise more!" is an almost impossible command. These plans often expect you to hurdle over the massive roadblocks of food addiction and toxic inflammation on sheer willpower alone. This is why most diets fail in the long run. You try to take the leap, but it's just too difficult. Then you feel filled with guilt and a sense of personal failure. You think less of yourself. And you give up.

I feel great empathy for the dieter in this situation. I've watched my patients helplessly struggle against an enemy that is bigger and stronger than they are. There is much prejudice in our culture against people who are overweight, and there is also a perception that they are somehow weak-willed, greedy, gluttonous, or lacking in strength of mind. This is completely unfair and untrue. Asking someone in a toxic inflammatory state to "just eat less and exercise more" is like asking someone with a broken leg to enter a dance contest. Or asking a drug addict to just stop doing drugs, or telling a clinically depressed person to snap out of it. You aren't just fighting your desire for a cookie; you are fighting against powerful internal biochemical forces. Your body doesn't want to stop consuming too many calories. Fat cells enclose toxins and protect you from them, which is why a toxic body quickly gains weight. Inflammation makes exercise hurt more. Your body is in panic mode, balanced in a precarious equilibrium in order to handle the onslaught of its current environment. Suddenly put it on a rigid diet and the demands are just too high. What if it needs to make more fat cells to protect you? What if burning those fat cells releases the toxins again into a body that isn't equipped to remove them? What if you don't eat the foods your gut bacteria now want? Your body is conserving energy to deal with these perceived threats, and that means less energy for you to live your life. Even if you win the battle and lose some weight, you are quite likely to lose the war and gain it back again.

Shifting the Scale

So what is your escape route? How do you get out of this biochemical prison? I know an ancient and secret passageway, a trapdoor, and your jailers can't do a thing about it. This secret passageway gives you the edge, biochemically and psychologically. This escape route works because it *primes your body* to succeed at making lifestyle changes by breaking the addiction cycle before you attempt to change one single thing—before you ever look at a meal plan or a calorie guide. If you prime your body for success by gently clearing the pathways in your body that eliminate waste, removing the accumulation of toxins, and slowly altering your gut bacteria in a direction that will call out for better choices, you will discover that lifestyle changes become easier. Weight loss, increased energy, and mental clarity will begin to happen *to you*, rather than you forcing them to happen. The way this works will feel pretty effortless, spontaneous. You won't have to rely on an impossible amount of willpower to begin changing your life.

Before I ever suggest that you should eat this or should not eat that, you will prime your body to beat me to the good advice. You will start changing. You will start moving more. You will start preferring foods that are good for you and encourage a healthy weight. You won't have to guilt yourself into skipping the cookie or the pizza. You won't want them as much, and you won't want as much of them. You will change because you want to, not because I told you to. This happens because as the toxins clear and the inflammation subsides, your body can slide gently into a newer, more stable equilibrium in which you will finally be able to feel for yourself what your body wants and what makes you feel great. You won't just achieve a lower number on the scale. You will achieve a whole new you: vigorous and energetic, mentally sharp and clearheaded, quick-thinking and full of life.

This is the purpose of *The Prime*: to prime your body and brain to function at the peak of health and wellness. Living a healthy life will feel awesome, not excruciating, because your body is primed for it. All you have to do is make a few easy changes on a schedule that is commensurate with your current level of health and toxicity (when you get to Chapter 6, you'll take a test to determine how fast you should move). You won't have to force yourself to comply with any dietary restrictions or give up one single thing you love—not dinner, not dessert, not any food group. Not even your sedentary lifestyle! In just a few weeks, your body will feel like a different one: Healthier. Sharper. Quicker. And thinner, too. No willpower required.

This book is the beginning of that education process. It is your defense, to keep you from falling prey to anyone's attempts to manipulate your choices again. I want to even the playing field because if the food you eat now is controlling your free will (and if you are overweight, this is likely), then you are probably not making independent and truly cognizant food choices. Once you regain control over your own biochemistry, however, you can regain control over your behavior. That's when you reclaim power.

Once we start voicing our biochemical free will, those companies—that are to a large extent responding to our demand, even if they helped create it—will change what they produce. This is already happening. For example, PepsiCo is buying up a lot of companies making healthy food. Walmart is selling organic produce. You can now find many healthy foods in the supermarket that were once only available at fringe-type health food stores.

But none of these positive trends help until *you* break free. Your biochemistry should be under your control, not the control of multinational corporations studying how to get you addicted. It's time to take back your life, your appetite, your mind, and your body.

In this book, I will demystify why we are eating the way we are eating from a biochemical, a neurological, and an Ayurvedic perspective. I will help you determine whether you are making decisions based on knowledge or based on addictive responses. Then I will show you exactly how to opt out of this codependent relationship with food.

And as for the food companies? It's a brilliant business model—you can't argue with it in those terms. You could even say it is the American dream: someone starts a company and uses science to increase profits astronomically until all the shareholders become fabulously wealthy. Our culture sanctions that kind of behavior . . . until we realize that we are the unwitting victims of it. Everything the processed food industry learns about how food works in the body, they have used to maximize their profits. Yes, America values profit. However, we value something else, too. We value free will, and free will is exactly what many people living and eating in the twenty-first century have lost.

I don't mind if companies try to be profitable, but I do mind having my free will taken away. Fortunately, you can reclaim food. You can fight biochemistry with biochemistry. Once you break the addiction cycle, you will want to choose foods that make you feel good rather than "high." This could even have a trickle-down effect that could improve the world: when enough people start making different kinds of food choices, this will send a clear message that food companies have to change, rather than manipulating us to conform to their bottom line. When we reclaim our biochemical free will, then we will be in a position to vote with our dollars about what kind of food we want available to us.

Are you ready to stop starting with the hardest part? Start easy, and weight loss, brain power, and boundless energy can be something your body does almost without effort. You just need to prepare it with The Prime.

What Is The Prime?

If The Prime doesn't tell you what to eat, what does it do? Let me explain this by way of an analogy. Doctors often use medications to treat issues for which that medicine is not labeled. This is called *off-label use*. We often find out by accident the unintended benefits of these medications after years of treating patients and observing the results. A seizure medication, for example, may happen to alleviate back pain. An antidepressant may coincidentally help treat nicotine addiction. A blood pressure medicine may, as a side effect, treat a tremor.

This is exactly what I am doing with The Prime. The program I put my patients on, to reduce their inflammation and toxin load and thereby begin to treat their neurological problems, had the unexpected side effect of causing spontaneous and sometimes dramatic weight loss. In essence, I am using my holistic neurology repair treatment program "off-label," to help you lose weight, even if you don't have a neurological problem. (And if you do? We'll be knocking out two problems with one effective approach.) This works because the same mechanisms that can cause neurological disturbances in the body can also cause weight gain. Correct those mechanisms, and the neurological disturbances as well as the weight problems can correct themselves.

This is why the program isn't really a diet. It's not exactly as simple as a detox, either. It is a subtle but intensive rebalancing of your system, to reduce inflammation, purge biochemical junk, restore a healthier mix of gut bacteria, repair digestion, and correct the biochemical processes that were keeping your body from maintaining a healthy, disease-free equilibrium. Putting your body back together, biochemically, is how you *prime* your body for a healthier life because the imbalances you are experiencing now are keeping you from practicing healthy habits. Once you right those biochemical wrongs, healthy habits won't just be easier to adopt. You will feel *compelled* to adopt them. This is why weight loss becomes practically effortless and spontaneous.

But weight loss isn't the only benefit you will see when you embark upon The Prime. You will also notice that you feel better. You have more energy. And, as you may have hoped when you saw that a neurologist wrote this book, you will probably notice some pretty dramatic improvement in any brain-related issues you may be having: headaches, brain fog, concentration issues, or forgetfulness. That's because The Prime isn't just encouraging weight loss. It's nudging your entire body toward health in a way that focuses on the digestive and neurological systems (and the interesting and complex interaction between them).

The Prime gives you body awareness so that you notice the subtle and not-so-subtle changes in the way you feel, think, and function according to what you eat. When this starts to happen, you will finally recognize that you may not want what you were eating and doing and thinking before. You may want something different, something healthier.

My patients feel this profoundly. As they go through my program, at first they get excited about their clothes fitting better and starting to feel more physically attractive, but that phase passes quickly. Soon, they get much more excited that their memory improves, their brain fog clears up, that making decisions is easier for them, that they have lost their tolerance for the negative things they used to put up with in life. They don't just feel better and look better. They get a clarity about their lives that they didn't have before, and then they start making real changes. The limits they thought applied to them no longer seem to apply. This is the most exciting part for me, too: to see my patients living at their prime.

In other words, although you will lose weight, what you gain may prove to be even more valuable to you: greater clarity, greater mental function, greater creativity, more energy, even more joy. Sure, it's fun to be able to fit into clothes you haven't worn in years. But honestly, I'm more interested in optimizing human potential.

I want to make it fun to be human again. I want it to feel good. I want you to be successful. For so many people, life and work and even eating have become oppressive, but life feels oppressive only because you are living in biochemical sewage. It's time to take out the trash.

How do we do it? We diet in reverse.

Let's go back to those early days in the clinic, when I first discovered that my neurological detoxification and anti-inflammatory program had the side effect of weight loss, so I can explain exactly how it works. The answer has one foot in modern Western medicine and one foot in the ancient science of Ayurveda.

As you learned in the Introduction, I have been trained in both conventional neurology and Ayurvedic medicine, and I use aspects of both systems in my treatment of neurology patients. Digestion is a key focus of Ayurveda and an important aspect of my treatment plan, but unlike many other diets you may have heard about, I don't start the work of improving digestion by changing what you are eating. In fact, I rarely mention many dietary changes to my patients when we first begin. Instead, I start them out by assessing their level of toxicity and inflammation. That determines how fast we go. I am a big proponent of a slower approach because I believe that slow and gradual changes have a more profound and lasting effect. Some patients don't have as much detoxifying to do, however, and can move along at a quicker pace. You'll take a quiz in Chapter 6 that will help you determine which track you will follow to move through each stage of the program:

- Fast Track, moving through each stage every two weeks
- Moderate Track, taking three weeks per stage
- Gentle Track, spending four weeks settling into each stage of the program, for steady, lasting changes in weight and brain function

The following are the four stages.

Stage One: Activate a Biochemical Shift

Stage One adds just four things to your daily routine to begin to shift your biochemistry. You don't have to take anything away:

1. Make a tea each morning made of cumin seeds, coriander seeds, and fennel seeds, and sip on it all day long. These simple ingredients have a profound detoxifying effect on the body.

2. Take 1 teaspoon each of ground flax seeds and psyllium husks every other night, mixed into a glass of room-temperature water. Fiber not only helps digestion by moving things along, but it carries out a lot of waste with it and has demonstrated anti-inflammatory effects.

3. Take triphala each night. Don't worry, it's nothing weird. Triphala is simply dried and ground-up berries: amlaki, bibhitaki, and haritaki. These are common elements used in cooking in India—everyone eats them.

4. Dry-brush your skin every day, preferably using special raw silk gloves. (I'll tell you exactly how to do this in Chapter 6.)

Stage Two: Crush Cravings (No Willpower Required!)

In Stage Two, you'll keep going with your Stage One habits, but I'll also give you strategies to curb the cravings that have you eating what you wish you wouldn't eat. We'll also be readjusting your gut bacteria, while infusing your body with nutrition that will support detoxification:

1. Add the gentle and powerful herb ashwagandha, for curbing sugar cravings and reducing the stress response.

2. Add another great herb called Brahmi, a serious brain booster that works to reverse neuroadaptation to addictive food components. (I'll tell you more about neuroadaptation in Chapter 3.)

3. Make and enjoy Prime Juice and Prime Broth, not to replace your regular meals but as an aid to fighting cravings when they strike.

4. Start a cravings journal. It's easy, and it won't take much time, I promise, but it will make a big difference in how you understand what you think you want to eat.

Stage Three: Ignite Energy and Fat

At this stage of the plan, you will add just a few more things and really get your body geared up to ignite fat and energize:

1. Try an herb made from the gum of the myrrh tree called guggul, one of the most powerful detoxifiers I know. Your digestion is going to start working better than you ever knew it could.

2. Learn how to make a homemade fat-burning curry powder you can add to your foods.

3. Make a simple preparation using ginger, lemon juice, and sea salt, to help stimulate your digestion before meals (I'll have a couple of other, less intense options, too, for those who prefer them). I'll tell you exactly who should use this Ginger Gut Flush and how often.

Stage Four: Biohack Your Lifestyle Habits

I'm still not going to tell you to stop eating anything you love, although by now, you may be feeling a little less love for the foods that have kept you captive, especially now that you are biochemically freed from them. In this chapter, however, I'm going to help you shift some things around and try a few strategies that can make a big difference in how you feel and how you choose to live:

1. Shift your meals around. Your largest meal is now at lunch. Seriously, you'll get used to this and thank me later.

2. Skip raw vegetables; they are now off the menu. It may sound counterintuitive, but trust me, this is one of the nicest things you can do for your digestion as it continues to heal (as we get into the program, I'll talk more about how long this will likely take for your individual situation). Also, warm drinks only. Forget that ice-cold glass of lemonade. Warm it up. Drink your water at room temperature. Easy, right?

3. Learn meditation—whatever method works for you. The effects of meditation on stress, cravings, and life improvement are well documented and profound.

4. Finally, be in bed by 10 p.m.! This may sound impossible if you are used to staying up late, but you can gradually downshift your bedtime until you're on target. This is the best way to take advantage of your body's natural repair and rejuvenation phases.

This is The Prime. After your four stages are complete, you will feel like a different person—newer, quicker, brighter, more energetic . . . and thinner. Only then will I give you some takeaways to help you transition from old habits to better ones, such as the best ways to cook, eat, and move for your individual and unique body system—if you want to go there. You can always go further if you feel inspired. The best part of The Prime is that it makes you supremely body-aware. You will feel when something doesn't agree with you, and you will sense when it does. You will know what your body really likes and wants and needs, what it thrives on, and what it doesn't. This is the true freedom The Prime offers you, and it's an exciting way to live.

CHAPTER 2

NOT YOUR EVERYDAY DETOX

One of the questions I get a lot is "Is The Prime a 'detox'?" To answer, it is important to explain some things about the way I perceive detoxification versus the way it is often talked about in the popular media. Throughout this book, I often mention that digestive dysfunction and consequential brain issues are the result of being in a toxic inflammatory state. But what does that mean, exactly?

You probably understand inflammation—you know what it looks like when you get an injury and it gets red and swollen. That happens inside your body, too, when you are exposed to injurious substances or actions. But *toxin* is a more nebulous word. You know it doesn't mean "poison," exactly. We're not talking about rat poison or arsenic (although in some cases we are talking about pesticides). So what is a "toxin" and what is a "detox"?

When we talk about toxins, what we are really talking about is *ama*.

All About Ama

Ama is the real target of The Prime. *Ama* is a word *sort of* like *toxin*, but it has a broader meaning. It is the Ayurvedic term for substances inside the body and mind that are insufficiently digested and/or are located in their current form in places they should not be—such as undigested proteins seeping through the lining of the gastro-intestinal (GI) tract or waste backing up and getting stuck in the lymphatic system or colon. Things that may be perfectly healthy somewhere in your body—such as a protein in your stomach or small intestine—become toxic when they get in the wrong place. Similarly, something that seems toxic, such as a pesticide or a drug, can become perfectly benign if your body is able to safely neutral-ize and eliminate it. Furthermore, ama can also be an undigested emotion in your psyche—a trauma from the past or an unresolved issue you can't think your way out of—that sits inside you. All of these things are ama.

MENTAL AMA

The idea that a "toxin" could be a physical substance or an emotion/thought is a difficult one for modern Western medi-cine to grasp. We have medical doctors and we have psycholo-gists, and these two don't necessarily confer or see problems in the same way. Their fields are often considered separately. However, in Ayurveda, these two fields are much more uni-fied. The Ayurvedic perspective does not distinguish be-tween toxins that are in the body and those that are in the mind. Ayurveda is concerned with toxins that are insufficiently transformed, whether in the body or in the mind, because this will do damage to the entire interconnected system. This ama eventually weakens both body and mind, resulting in disease.

The Detox: Purging Ama

The whole point of a "detox" in my world is to get ama out of the system. Some detoxes and cleanses you may encounter do this, even if they don't use that terminology, but others don't help at all, or even make the situation worse. Unfortunately, words like *detox* and *cleanse* are buzzwords that are often misused, and there is a lot of confusion and misinformation about the concept of detoxification.

Some health professionals, including many doctors, tell you that it is completely unnecessary to "detox" or "cleanse" because the digestive tract completely sheds and rebuilds its lining every few days,[1] and because the body has powerful natural detoxification systems that take care of most problems. Other health professionals advocate periodic "detoxes" or "cleanses," even those that are quite extreme and devoid of calories and nutrients. But whether you are a detox or cleanse aficionado or one of those people who think subsisting on green juice for three days would be nothing short of torture, I want you to understand that the truth is somewhere in the middle. Extreme cleanses, especially without any physical and mental preparation, can be not just unpleasant but harmful to the body. They release toxins too quickly, without providing much if any nutrition, and they deprive the body of energy. This deprivation can cause you to lose lean muscle mass and trigger extreme cravings, undoing any detoxification or benefit that might have happened.

The idea that we don't need to cleanse or detoxify at all to be healthy, however, is simply untrue. Our bodies do have natural detoxification systems in place—effective ones that work hard all the time. When your body encounters toxic elements in the air you breathe, in the water you drink, in the foods you eat, from exposure to viruses and bacteria, or even from the by-products of our own metabolism, it has to do something so it is not injured by them. It has to protect itself. This happens in several important ways that impact (and sometimes interfere with) digestion:

- By eliminating toxins through the digestive system, including through the liver and colon and through the kidneys and bladder.

- By eliminating toxins through the sweat glands and the lungs. This happens continuously.

- By storing the toxins in fat cells, where they are sealed away (until that fat is burned). This is a major reason why toxicity often contributes directly to excess body fat. If your body can't remove the toxin before it can hurt you, the safest solution is to store it safely away in your fat cells. The body will keep pumping it into your fat cells, until the fat cells can no longer accommodate the toxic load.

- By storing toxins in the organs. This causes inflammation due to the irritation and can also trigger an autoimmune response. When circulating or embedded toxins resemble tissues in our own bodies (something called *molecular mimicry*), the body may attempt to eliminate the pathogen by attacking not just the foreign substance but the body cells it resembles. This can eventually result in autoimmune disease, as our own immune system aggressively destroys our bodies in an attempt to get to the perceived toxin. Many new fields are investigating how toxins can disrupt normal biochemistry when they are stored within an organ. In fields such as functional medicine and endobiogeny (a systems-theory approach to the body's internal workings, which I believe will be the next wave in medicine in another decade), we are discovering new methods of early detection of autoimmunity. This is just another example of how science is exploring ahead of medical education. It is an exciting area of research!

- Finally, your body eliminates mental and emotional toxins through a variety of thought processes, especially when you deliberately attempt to work things out and address personal issues, but also in less obvious ways, like burying traumas in the subconscious (in much the same way the body buries toxins in fat cells, to keep them from harming you). Meditation becomes a crucial process in The Prime for facilitating the elimination of emotional and mental waste products.

MODERN ENVIRONMENTAL TOXINS

The world is filled with more environmental toxins than at any other time in history. When an organism (such as a person) absorbs a toxic substance, such as a pesticide or a drug or some other environmental chemical, what should happen is *biotransformation*. This is the process by which the body transforms a substance, such as a nutrient, a drug, or a chemical, into a different form, often for absorption or safe elimination by the body. If your body can't handle the toxic load, and you absorb the toxins faster than you can process them out of the body, then you will experience *bioaccumulation*. This is how mercury builds up in fish, and how heavy metals, pesticides, PCBs, dioxins, and other chemicals build up inside you. Your body has to store them if they can't be processed.

Here are some of the toxins your body has to contend with today:

• We have created or isolated and released over 100,000 toxic chemicals[2] into our environment—into the air, the water, and the food we eat. We have barely begun to study all of these for their effects on humans. Less than 5 percent of them have even been studied for human safety!

• A study by the Environmental Working Group found an average of two hundred industrial chemicals and pollutants in the cord blood of newborn babies in the United States. Toxins found in newborn cord blood included pesticides; perfluorochemicals used as stain and oil repellants in fast-food packaging, clothing, and textiles; Teflon chemicals; flame retardants; pollutants from burning coal and gasoline; and many toxins present in common consumer products.[3]

- Every day, about fifteen thousand new chemicals are registered on the American Chemical Society's chemicals list, according to an article from the Science + Technology newsletter out of UC Santa Barbara.[4]

- Every year, industry releases approximately ten million tons of toxic chemicals into the environment.[5]

- Artificial sweeteners have been shown to be carcinogenic and neurotoxic.

- High-fructose corn syrup increases the kind of cholesterol that increases the risk of heart disease and diabetes.

- Trans fats have been linked to increasing harmful LDL cholesterol and decreasing helpful HDL cholesterol.

- Monosodium glutamate and other flavorings can trigger headaches and other neurological disturbances.

- Preservatives such as sulfites, nitrates and nitrites, BHA, and BHT have a wide range of known negative effects on health.

- Chemicals can be found in most of the products that we use every day—not just in foods, but also in personal care products, cleaning products, makeup, utensils, water and baby bottles, carpet, paint, furniture, gardens and lawns, vehicles, and the houses and other buildings inside which we spend most of our time living or working. For example, one study showed that the plastic bags made for roasting chickens impart endocrine disruptors into the food.[6]

As you can see, toxins cause more problems than tight pants and low energy—they can create disease. These systems are all crucial for survival (even the mental and emotional detoxification systems). However, we live in a highly toxic environment, and our bodies need a little help. When the toxic load from modern living overwhelms the body's natural detoxification systems, which were never meant to handle the onslaught of so much pollution, processed food, and such a sedentary lifestyle, we need to intervene to prevent the development of chronic disease and brain dysfunction.

Signs of Ama

Ama may not be measurable by Western science yet, but Ayurveda teaches that it is something you can recognize because it manifests in the body through obvious physical signs and symptoms. Some of these are the following:

- **Ama has a foul odor.** Ama doesn't stink when inside your body, but when it mixes with excretory products such as sweat, urine, and stool as they are expelled from the body, it develops a strong and unpleasant smell. Because ama has this smell, people often complain that they develop an unpleasant smell while doing a detox. Whenever I detox, my sweat develops what I call my "funk smell" in my right armpit. You may also notice that while doing The Prime, your urine and stool begin to smell stronger and more unpleasant than before. If they stink now, ama is already seeping out of you and you definitely need to detox! Perhaps surprisingly, a healthy person with a low ama load will have sweat, urine, and even stool that don't have a foul smell. In fact, when I am not detoxing, I don't need to wear deodorant at all.
- **Ama is sticky.** Because ama is sticky, when you are secreting a lot of ama into your stool, you can experience constipation.

The stool doesn't want to move. It wants to stick to your insides like caramel on a spoon. This is also why constipation often happens at the beginning of a detox. This can make people believe the detox isn't working because they feel all clogged up, but it means the detox *is* working because the ama is coming out. It just needs a little help. Fiber is the answer here—it sweeps up the ama from your gut and moves it out more easily. (This is an important part of The Prime.) The stickiness of ama can also contribute to skin breakouts during a detox because ama clogs the pores. If you have constipation and adult acne before you start a detox, you can be pretty sure ama is the culprit.

- **Ama makes you tired.** Ama produces lethargy in the body. It can even make you feel like you are wading through water all the time. People who are detoxing often feel tired at first as the toxins start to move out of the body. If you battle fatigue and lethargy now, you probably already have excess ama.

- **Ama leads to weight gain and chronic disease.** This is an interesting avenue of research in my opinion: weight gain that causes chronic disease is not so much about excess calories. It is more about excess toxic calories. A recent study attempted to show that obesity caused diabetes, and although the researchers found that these two states were associated, they could not prove causation. They could not prove that being obese caused diabetes. However, they could measure GGT, which strongly correlated with a diabetic state. To simplify, GGT is an indirect measure of a person's toxic exposure. The study found that when GGT was elevated and an individual was overweight, there was a strong correlation with diabetes.[7] Toxicity combined with weight gain is linked to the formation of diabetes. It's not just excessive calorie consumption alone that causes the problem. Some people are overweight and do not have diabetes because they are not in a toxic inflammatory state. They do not have a backup of ama. Consider artificial sweeteners—toxic but without calories. They have been linked to obesity[8] and also to diabetes.[9] This is an example of ama causing its damage.

Why Your Doctor May Not Think You Need to Detox

This brings us to another big issue. Maybe you are all ready to jump in and detox, clearing the ama from your system, and that's great—until you tell your doctor about it. A few doctors may be on board with your plan—especially integrative physicians (physicians who work with healing methods from many different traditions, like Ayurveda, traditional Chinese medicine, functional medicine, endobiogeny, chiropractic care, and naturopaths). These doctors may have already received training about how toxins (ama) build up, and what to do about it. Many other doctors, however—especially those who are conventionally trained—may be less supportive of the concept of detox. I know because I used to be one of those doctors.

The reason many Western doctors don't understand the purpose of detoxing is largely a matter of terminology. In Western medicine, the word *toxic* has a specific meaning. It is a critical state resulting from a life-threatening accumulation of poisons, from either a drug (such as acetaminophen), an intoxicating substance (such as alcohol or heroin), or an infection (such as in the case of toxic shock). In Western medicine, we are trained to think of this not as part of a chronic disease process, but rather as an acute state. *Toxic* means you get to the hospital, *stat!*

So when you go in to your doctor's office and complain of "toxins" or suggest you need a "cleanse," your doctor hears something different from what you mean. You and your doctor are talking about two completely different things. You are using the same word, *toxin*, to describe totally separate problems. And while ama is not a medical emergency, its eventual result in the body, if it is not removed or dealt with, could turn into a medical tragedy. You are right to want to do something about it.

But the problem lies with the information lag between conventional Western medicine and integrative medicine. Those of us who practice in both modes (Western and integrative) like to think that science will soon catch up with more progressive health systems. However, Western medicine isn't really set up for this yet. When Western scientists demand quantitative proof of the direct cause of a condition (such as a toxic, inflammatory state) before determining a treatment, it becomes necessary for them to hyperfocus on one specific symptom or condition, rather than look at the whole system as it works together. This is a limited view with slow results.

Even once we know something is "true" as supported by rigorous scientific research, it won't be a part of a medical school curriculum for decades. Actually, modern scientists know quite a lot—much more than is currently practiced in most medical clinics. Medical information doubles every three years. (I've seen estimates that by 2020, the volume of medical data will double every three days!) Yet it is an extremely long process to get something from the research stage into the medical curriculum and then into clinical practice, and this creates a massive information lag in medicine that we have never seen before. For this reason, what a student currently learns in medical school is already largely outdated by the time that same student begins to practice medicine. We've never known this much and not practiced it!

I believe this phenomenon is responsible for the perceived rift between the way medicine is traditionally taught, and integrative approaches that have chosen to jump ahead and take a look at the rising mountain of data on lifestyle medicine and start integrating some of that information into clinical care *now*. For example, the Institute of Functional Medicine has made it a priority to take newly created data coming out of the scientific research community and figure out ways to use the data now, before it has to spend decades trickling down the conventional chain of knowledge and into the standard of care for medical practice.

One unfortunate side effect of this situation is a lot of finger pointing. Conventional doctors believe they are the ones practicing evidence-based medicine because the information has been vetted over the course of decades. They say, "I'm right because I'm practicing what I learned in medical school and it is proven." Integrative physicians, on the other hand, believe they are the ones practicing evidence-based medicine because they are working with data that is coming out of molecular biology, genetics, and nutritional medicine—data that is cutting-edge, current, and being released *right now*. They say, "I'm right because I am practicing what is new, rather than what is old and outdated." Here we have a massive tug-of-war, and the patient is caught in the middle, unsure which side to choose and wondering, "Who's right?" The problem is, they both are.

Both sides are right, based on the information they are using, and there are arguments for the tried-and-true just as there are arguments for the brand-new. One family practice doctor may be using information and effective techniques he learned in medical school twenty-five years ago, while another (and I consider myself one of these) is using information that will be taught in medical schools twenty-five years from now. We are both right, but at different times in history.

Normally, the old ways die off over the course of centuries, but information is coming to us at such a fast and furious rate in the modern world that two different "rights" can now exist at the same time. This has never happened before.

What does this mean for you? Right now, patients are living in a sort of medical dual reality, and so are doctors. Who is right depends on which question is being asked.

But let me give you some guidance:

1. If the question is "Which medications can treat my current symptoms?" then your conventional doctor's answer is likely right.

2. If the question is "How do I get off medications and reverse this disease process?" then your integrative doctor's answer is likely right.

What is interesting is that as some of this information on life-style medicine is becoming more mainstream, such as the role of gluten in autoimmune disease, of meditation in the treatment of cardiovascular disease, or of sugar in heart disease, my colleagues who thought I was practicing "voodoo" before now come up to me and say, "Oh yeah, I guess that is right after all ... *now*." As if it hadn't been right before. Yet they have a valid point in that it is finally being proven and supported by enough people within the medical field that they feel comfortable accepting it as true *now*. I just wasn't comfortable waiting any longer when I became a patient and saw the problem from the other side of the stethoscope.

I want you to understand the big picture of modern medicine because I hope it will help explain a lot of the confusion and frustration that patients and doctors are feeling. Sometimes my patients come to me and say, "Why didn't my regular doctor tell me this stuff? Why is my regular doctor not on my side?" Conventional doctors are *not* against you, they are just practicing what they know. I, on the other hand, am practicing what I know—ironically, a lot of it is knowledge that has been around for five thousand years but is only now becoming proven, bit by bit, according to Western scientific standards.

I understand that this is frustrating for everyone. Many doctors are uncomfortable recommending anything they haven't learned about in medical school or continuing education. Many patients don't want to know how uncertain the science on which medical decisions are based really is. But this uncertainty is a reality. We continue to learn, and there is much we do not know yet. If you are okay with that uncertainty, this will provide for a huge amount of personal freedom, as well as personal responsibility. It puts your health back into your hands. It shifts the focus from what your doctor is writing on a prescription pad to what you are putting at the end of your fork.

So here's the bottom line: if you don't detoxify (and by that I mean, if you do not do something to clear out excess, built-up ama in your body and mind), you will have a much harder time losing weight, resolving your neurological issues, and regaining energy, vibrancy, and health. If you clear out the ama periodically, you will strengthen the natural detox pathways in your body and provide it with the micronutrients it needs to fully use these systems. This makes weight loss, mental clarity, and health much easier to attain.

AMA: CLUES IN WESTERN MEDICINE

Although there is not a clear Western equivalent to ama, I believe it is coming. I am most excited by recent developments in the field of molecular toxicology, which is the study of the effects of chemicals on living organisms. I predict that within the next decade, we will have a clearer scientific perspective on what ama is and how it works in the body on multiple levels. Studies in this field are demonstrating how even small doses of toxic substances can result in chronic cellular dysfunction. These doses can be in nanograms (a nanogram is one billionth of a gram, or 1/1,000,000,000—an inconceivably small amount). This is toxicity at the cellular level, and is completely different from the kind of toxins I was trained to identify in medical school (such as acute alcohol toxicity or acetaminophen toxicity). I believe that this line of research will "discover" ama with a molecular definition that will finally help all physicians understand its importance. This may even allow Western medicine to refine the Ayurvedic concept of ama by discovering molecular subcategories of ama, or different ways ama manifests in the body biochemically. This will also help mainstream science better understand how to deal with it, adding credence and scientific specificity to Ayurveda's ancient knowledge about a phenomenon that plagues so many people in the modern world.

So is The Prime a detox? The answer is yes—and no. It will have a profound detoxification effect on your system, but it probably is unlike any detox you've ever done before. That's because it shifts deeply rooted ama from your body and mind; that's what The Prime is really about.

But what ama does in the body is complex and impacts your life in many ways. To fully understand this, and to give you the motivation you need to embrace The Prime and change your body, I want you to understand what's going on in your brain, your belly, and your entire body. I want you to understand the science and why The Prime is so much more than a detox—it is a biochemical paradigm shift backed by solid research and results. I want you to see why, on a real, cellular level, The Prime will change you.

PART TWO

Prime Science

CHAPTER 3

NEUROADAPTATION, FOOD ADDICTION, AND YOUR BRAIN

The brain adapts to its environment. This ability is one of the brain's most impressive and life-sustaining characteristics. Change the brain's environment, and the brain changes in response. This process is called *neuroadaptation*, and as a neurologist I find it one of the most fascinating things about the brain—and one of the most frustrating. If you are struggling with food addiction, if you have excess weight on you, or if you feel like your brain isn't performing at its peak, one of the main reasons is neuroadaptation.

Neuroadaptation is a complex and useful brain function, but it also causes us a lot of trouble in the modern world, and it is the primary reason why you may not have been able to stick to a diet in the past. When I say you are dieting backward, I mean that you are fighting an uphill battle against neuroadaptation; until you set your brain's internal environment right, you will have a much more difficult—even impossible—time attempting to change anything in your external environment, and that includes lifestyle changes you want to make, such as dieting and exercise. I want The Prime to work for you, and for that to happen, you need to understand why what you are doing now isn't working—and why what I am going to ask you to do will.

What Is Neuroadaptation?

Neuroadaptation is the brain's amazing ability to adapt to whatever you do to your body. Eat a lot of sugar? Your brain adapts, finding a new equilibrium that makes allowances for sugar. Drink a lot of coffee? Your brain adapts. Take drugs? Your brain adapts. Exercise daily? Your brain adapts. Live with chronic stress? Your brain adapts. That adaptation may be precarious—an uneasy, relatively unsteady equilibrium called *allostasis*—but your brain knows that it can function to keep you alive if you keep changing the rules of the game.

But neuroadaptation can work for or against us. You can see how it works against us in the case of drug dependence. Many illegal drugs and also alcohol cause the brain to release dopamine, which induces feelings of pleasure. Many pleasurable things trigger the release of dopamine, but drugs and alcohol trigger a much larger dopamine response, causing more intense pleasure than, for example, a snack of sweet grapes or a walk in the park on a nice day. To your brain, this flood of dopamine isn't normal and it perceives the situation as stressful, even if the feeling is pleasurable to the person experiencing it. If this extreme pleasure is repeated often enough (such as with habitual drug use or drinking), your brain adjusts to create a more normal, stable environment for itself again, by switching off some of your dopamine receptors. When this happens, you won't be able to use or feel all that dopamine anymore because you have fewer receptors to receive it. Your brain is adapting to blunt the pleasure response it perceives as abnormal and stressful. This is why the same amount of drug or alcohol eventually becomes less pleasurable. That is the brain's goal, but it isn't always an effective long-term strategy because this usually doesn't cause the person to stop using the drug or alcohol—it only makes him or her use more, which causes more dopamine receptors to go offline. Now the user can't feel as much pleasure with anything, so even if he or she quits the drug or alcohol, everything feels worse.

Even those grapes and that nice walk in the park don't give the pleasure they did before the drug or alcohol use, because there are fewer dopamine receptors in operation. This causes bad feelings—withdrawal symptoms.

Doctors see this all the time with pain medication. We give patients a certain amount, and their need for it only increases because of this brain receptor downregulation. The same amount of medication doesn't provide the same amount of pain relief anymore. That's because the neurotransmitter release from the medication was too extreme, and the body reacted to this stressful change in its brain chemistry by decreasing those receptors. We also see this with Parkinson's drugs that stimulate the dopamine receptors. When a patient has been taking these medications for long periods, the drug gets less and less effective and neurologists have to continue increasing the doses.

This isn't a book about drug addiction, but perhaps you have already extrapolated that drugs and alcohol are not the only substances that have this addictive effect. Tobacco and caffeine do, but so do certain foods. If you have ever wondered whether you are "addicted" to sugar or fat or cheese or junk food, you were on the right track. In fact, many food substances, especially those in type and quantity far removed from their natural forms (i.e., highly processed), have a neurological impact quite similar to the impact of a drug. They create an extreme pleasure response—more extreme than you should get from food—and the brain responds accordingly by adjusting to the perceived stress of too much pleasure.

To your brain, a candy or French fry binge doesn't feel all that different from a cocaine binge or a morphine injection. They even look similar on a PET scan (a type of imaging that allows doctors to look at organs and tissues), lighting up the same parts of the brain. In someone who is very overweight, the brain similarities are even more striking. This is because in people who are obese, neuroadaptation to sugar has already taken place in much the same way neuroadaptation to cocaine takes place. The addicted brain looks the same.

THE HPA AXIS

Stress affects the body through a process involving the HPA axis. *HPA* stands for the links between three central glands in the body that manage stress: the hypothalamus, the pituitary gland, and the adrenal glands. When the brain perceives stress, it signals the hypothalamus to release corticotrophin-releasing hormone (CRF), which binds to receptors on the pituitary gland. This signals the pituitary to release adrenocorticotropic hormone (ACTH), which binds to receptors on the adrenal glands. This in turn causes the adrenal glands to release cortisol, a steroid hormone that causes multiple physical stress-response effects in the body. Combined, these allow you to run faster, jump higher, and react more quickly. They interfere with digestion (because nobody is enjoying a nice meal during an emergency) and send blood to your muscles and heighten your senses.

This is meant to be a short-term situation. As soon as cortisol reaches a certain concentration in your bloodstream (giving you enough time to react appropriately to the stressor, such as jumping back on the curb to get out of the way of a speeding car or finishing your speech in front of the board of directors), the adrenals send the "all clear" signal, telling the hypothalamus and the pituitary to stop releasing CRF and ACTH. Eventually the cortisol works its way out of your bloodstream, you calm down, and your body returns to its normal, nonstressed state—a balanced state called *homeostasis*.

However, when your body stays stressed for too long or gets stressed too often (which can happen in the case of addiction), you lose your sensitivity to cortisol's signals. Your hypothalamus and pituitary keep telling your adrenals to produce cortisol until they are exhausted and you end up with a constant supply of cortisol in your bloodstream at a higher level than is normal. You get strung out and your body, always neuroadapting, tries to make the best of a bad situation. It achieves a new sort of balance by altering your brain chemistry (and even your behavior), but it is a detrimental balance that can lead to health issues. This is called *allostasis*, or the state of having adapted to a chronic stressor by making physical and chemical changes in the body. It is stable-ish, but less stable than homeostasis. I would even go so far as to call it a pre-disease state.

Neuroadaptation was never built for survival in our modern world. When the cookies, cheeseburgers, or tequila don't satisfy the way they did, we seek *more, more, more.* We want that pleasure back, and now the same things that gave it to us before don't cut it anymore because now we are short on dopamine receptors. We are at war with the brain—we want one thing (to feel good) and the brain wants something completely different (to create a stable environment so it can function).

It may sound incredible that food could do this. It's not Parkinson's medication. It's not pain medication. It's not heroin or meth or a bottle of Scotch. And yet it is basically having the same effect. Food, the way it is processed today, is simply too strong for the body and mind. It's too intense, in an unhealthy way, and when I say *unhealthy* I mean much more than just a lack of nutrients or too many calories or artificial ingredients. I mean that food alters your brain function. That great buzz you get from high-sugar, high-fat foods, whether pizza or cheese doodles or chocolate chip cookies, is causing your brain to pare back its dopamine receptors, and then the sugar and fat don't make you feel as good anymore, and you have to have more. Result: addiction. Studies have shown that people who are extremely overweight, as well as addicts and alcoholics, have significantly fewer dopamine receptors than non-addicts.[1] This is neuroadaptation, working in the only way it knows how to keep you alive and functioning.

And just as with drugs or alcohol, if you try to quit the addictive substance—the sugar or fat or junk food or alcohol or drugs or whatever it is—you are left not only with no pleasure-inducing substances, but with hardly any dopamine receptors, either. That means things that give healthy non-addicted people pleasure (such as small amounts of sweet things or fatty things or a glass of wine or a night of romance) suddenly don't do anything for you anymore. Guess what happens when you try to go on a diet? Withdrawal symptoms. This causes misery, pain, depression, and a strong urge for relief. You want the pleasure back, but now it's not even about pleasure anymore—it's about relieving pain and just trying to feel normal. You want to feel the way you used to feel, back before you ever started eating or drinking or doing the thing that gave you the initial high—and the only way you know how to feel any better is by doing more of the same thing. It's the only thing that gives relief. This is why so many addicts relapse.

WHAT IS ADDICTION?

According to the *DSM-IV* (the *Diagnostic and Statistical Manual of Mental Disorders*), which sets the criteria for how to classify every type of psychological problem, a person is addicted if he or she shows at least three of these seven symptoms. Although the manual does not specifically list food as an addictive substance, I have added my own comments to show you how easily food fits into the addiction model. As you read this, replace the word *substance* with *food* (or with those particular foods you can't stop eating) and see how it resonates with you:

1. The person is unable to cut down on substance use despite attempts.

   I see this a lot. People continually turn to food to deal with stress or unpleasant feelings, even if they know they are overeating and it is harming their health and negatively impacting their lifestyle.

2. The person consumes more substance than he or she intended.

     This is frequent with people who binge on food.

3. The person spends a lot of time getting the substance, using the substance, and recovering from the effects of the substance.

     This happens when people obsess about food, binge on food, and then feel the need to recover.

4. The more the person uses a substance over time, the more it takes of the substance to produce the desired effect.

     This is the result of those decreased dopamine receptors I told you about. This is proven to happen in people who are overweight.

5. The person gives up old activities with friends and family members in favor of the substance.

     This often happens when people are ashamed of their eating or bingeing. They pick at salads in public and then overeat in private.

6. The person experiences withdrawal, or physiological or psychological effects of stopping the substance.

     These are essentially detoxification symptoms. Everybody will experience them when stopping an addictive substance and even The Prime will include some detox symptoms, but they will be much milder than with a cold-turkey approach.

7. Negative consequences have no effect on the pattern of use.

     This is perhaps one of the most dramatic things I see with food addictions. Even though people are developing chronic diseases that will shorten their lives, they can't stop overeating or making food choices they know are harming them. They are miserable being overweight, but they can't stop eating things such as high-sugar and high-fat foods just to feel normal.

Fortunately, all is not lost, even if you feel hopelessly addicted to doughnuts or bacon or margaritas. You can retrain your dopamine receptors, switching them back on again. They can normalize and you *can* feel the way you used to feel. It takes time and a purposeful process, however. If you are "clean" for about twelve months, you have a high chance of staying that way because the brain has adapted back to a normal state, and if you have tools to help you stay clean without so much effort, you can accomplish this. (And if twelve months seems too long for you to wait, fear not—The Prime will start making noticeable changes right away. It's just that for most people, it takes twelve months to get all the way back.) While there will always be a memory of that escalated dopamine response—which is why people who are addicted to drugs, alcohol, or a food substance such as refined sugar often relapse if they have even a little bit of the offending pleasurable substance—the allure will steadily weaken the more you rebuild your health and brain strength. You will get "addicted" (in a healthy way) to feeling good and strong and in control of your own behavior. Doesn't that sound nice?

Neuroadaptation and Your Diet

Eating should feel good. The only reason you may be struggling with it now is that you are in an allostatic state. Allostasis is like homeostasis, but more precarious—the balance your brain creates under stressful circumstances. The problem is not the neuroadaptation but the environment we have created for ourselves, and our brain's efforts to survive in it. Now that so much of our food is junk, processed food, we are constantly faced with a delectable mixture of sugar, salt, and fat in amounts much higher than occur in any natural food. In junk food, those substances, so necessary for our survival, are no longer in anything close to natural proportions or natural forms. Junk food takes sugar and salt and fat *way too far*. It is sugar on steroids, fat to the max, the saltiest salt. It is food transformed (biochemically, at least) into an addictive drug.

THE SILVER LINING OF NEUROADAPTATION

Neuroadaptation may sound like something you wish didn't exist, but in actuality, we should all be grateful for it. Although it sometimes has effects that can be hard on us when we over-indulge, its original purpose was to encourage us to do things that enhanced our survival. Craving sugar is a good thing in an environment where humans have to seek out ripe fruit that isn't available year-round—we have to get it when we can get it. Craving fat is a good thing when the body needs fat for brain function or warmth and there are ripe avocadoes or coconuts hanging on the trees, or when winter is coming and humans need to hunt heavy, rich animal food in order to survive. Craving salt is a good thing because it helps maintain electrolyte balance in the body and can help prevent dehydration in times of water scarcity. Neuroadaptation encourages survival of the species. When we do something good for us, such as move around or eat an avocado or a pear or have sex, the brain releases a nice little shot of dopamine, so we feel good and want to do it some more. More exercise. More fruit. More love. In the days when things such as natural sugar and fat and potential mates were hard to come by, neuroadaptation gave us a nice little boost to seek those things out.

Worse yet, it is always available and cheap in any season, making it hard to avoid or resist. There is no "get it while you can" situation anymore. Today, people still enjoy things like ripe fruit and avocadoes and coconuts and animal meat and healthful salts like natural sea salt. These things still light up our pleasure centers, but not nearly to the extent that more extreme versions of these tastes do. The signals that were there to help ensure your survival are running amok. They're so overstimulated that, instead of getting this gentle little dopamine response that says, "Hey, you may want to eat a little bit more of this because these fruits are going to be out of season" or "You better feast on that buffalo because we don't know when you're going to get your next dose of fat," you are getting these massive spikes, and on a regular basis. It won't happen if you have a few bites of chocolate now and then, the occasional cookie or handful of French fries, but in the amounts many people eat these foods (because their bodies tell them they want more, more, more), the spike is extremely stressful to your physiology and especially to your neurochemistry. It feels good, in a crazy unstable way, and it's easy to get that "high."

Overeating pleasurable foods causes stress, but once you are caught in that stress loop, outside stressors can trigger a return to the thing that gives you pleasure, further exacerbating the stress. Some people are particularly vulnerable to this—childhood trauma can make your HPA axis more susceptible to stimulation, and emotional upheaval in the present moment (that wedding, that divorce, that new job or new baby) can also make you more susceptible to behaviors that seem to temporarily reduce stress (but actually increase it), such as drinking too much alcohol or overeating. How you feel and what happens to you has a direct impact on your biochemistry, and without acknowledging this, you will have a much more difficult time succeeding at positive health changes if other areas of your life are unstable.

An interesting 2002 article in *Nature Neuroscience* discussed a study of social dominance in monkeys who could self-administer cocaine. When monkeys were put together in a social housing situation, the dominant monkeys increased their dopamine receptors naturally and were less likely to self-administer cocaine. Submissive monkeys had no increase in dopamine receptors in response to the new housing and were more likely to self-administer cocaine, apparently as a coping mechanism. The study concluded that environmental changes can cause profound biological shifts that result in behavioral alterations, including vulnerability to addiction. Because this study involved animals, and willpower was not a factor, it clearly demonstrates the power of both biochemistry and stress in addictive behaviors.

It's a sad fact that even though food addiction is every bit as real as drug addiction, doctors and other health experts typically don't treat it that way. The attitude is that the overweight person should "just stop overeating." Yet if you don't take into account the biochemistry that's in place, that's simply an impossible request, one that only makes people feel worse and increases stress and isolation, thus compounding the problem.

Maybe you think this isn't you. Maybe your life is pretty well under control. You feel okay. You aren't *that* overweight, and you sure as hell aren't going to give up your evening glass of wine and your cheese or cookies or whatever it is you like. Because they help you cope (or so you think). But here's what I know from my clinic experience: If you can't lose weight or if you are overweight, you have this addiction. If you feel chronically tired or cloudy or have a hard time concentrating, you have this addiction. If you can't stop eating something because it makes you feel better (for a while), you have this addiction. Food is the biggest addiction in our nation. It is not rare. It happens easily. And it is nothing to be ashamed of. We can fix it.

Maybe now you better understand what you thought was your own lack of willpower. Giving in to cravings and addictive responses is just an attempt to escape the biochemical muck you have inadvertently created by repeatedly escaping through your pleasure response. This is why my patients say to me, "I don't know why I'm eating this. I don't know why I'm doing this to myself." You watch someone with an addiction and you may think, "But your liver is dying and you have gastric ulcers. Why are you still drinking?" or "But you are morbidly obese with type 2 diabetes and high blood pressure and arteriosclerosis. Why are you still overeating?" The answer is easy: These people (and you may be one of them) are using the only way they know to escape the high-stress environment they are in—a situation they often created inadvertently by using the substance (food, drink, drugs) to escape stress initially. Now they are no longer seeking pleasure, but rather a feeling of normalcy. The substance use has become a small, temporary, ineffective relief, but it is the only relief available. It's no wonder alcoholics and drug addicts and food addicts can't "just stop."

DOCTORS TAKE NOTE

I want to make this point strongly to both those who struggle with weight issues and the health professionals who treat them: this is a biochemical phenomenon. Would a doctor tell a diabetic, "What is wrong with you? Just don't let your blood sugar get too high. Make more insulin!" Would a doctor tell an alcoholic or a drug addict, "Just stop drinking" or "Just quit the heroin already"? Of course not. If it were that simple, nobody whose life was getting destroyed by addiction would ignore that advice. Instead, for addicts, there are long inpatient programs that are closely monitored because the biochemistry of a drug addiction is potentially deadly. Anyone who has had a loved one with an addiction problem knows firsthand what a strong hold addiction can have on the body and the mind.

We need to approach food addictions with far more compassion than we currently do. It's particularly difficult to treat food addictions because it's socially acceptable to overeat and eat junk food. And unlike any other substance, junk food is advertised everywhere. Imagine seeing a billboard for 99 cent heroin! We've made addictive food so readily available and so cheap that it's not only unfair but cruel. What's more, for a physician, I believe it is unprofessional and even unethical to look an overweight patient in the eye and tell him or her that the problem can be solved with willpower. When I think about the phenomenal patients I've seen, I know that their food addictions don't take away from who they are. They simply have a biochemical problem. We are marginalizing people without taking into consideration the cause of their supposed infraction!

I don't know why physicians don't use the humane approaches that have been proven so effective in treating other recognized addictions. When the patient in front of you feels acceptance and compassion, it directly helps relieve the stress response, and that makes changing destructive habits just a little bit easier. It does nothing to say, "But it's so easy to eat less; and your life depends on it." Shaming isn't good for anyone on a human level, and it makes change even more difficult. People who are shamed withdraw. They get so tired of being judged that they hide from the world and nurse their pleasure centers in isolation. Until doctors and other health professionals can stop shaming and judging and start helping patients overcome the biochemistry and psychology of the addiction cycle, there is no dialogue. This doesn't help patients heal.

How The Prime Works with, Not Against, Neuroadaptation

You can power through a diet like a drug addict in rehab, but the sad fact is that most addicts relapse, even after getting clean. Dieters are no different. Unless . . . unless you ease your brain out of its adaptive state slowly and gently, coaxing those dopamine surges to get a little bit slower and a little bit lower, until they are back to where they should be for appropriate responses to healthful food without ever making you too uncomfortable. Working with instead of against neuroadaptation means there is no stress and trauma related to withdrawal. When detoxification from addictive substances (no matter what they are) is a gradual process, the brain can adjust in a way that feels much less painful.

This is what The Prime does. It is a back-door method to thwart the dependency-related aspects of neuroadaptation. Here's why:

The Prime Downregulates the Stress Response

First, we will downregulate the stress response so the pleasure spikes from food become weaker triggers to activate the dopamine pathway. There are many ways we do this. One of the chief strategies is through an herb called ashwagandha, which is one of my most powerful tools for calming the brain. Food can be your ally, too. For example, you can add certain things to your foods that will calm the craving response you get from more stimulating foods. Natural salt (especially mineral-rich Himalayan salt) instead of regular table salt, ghee (clarified butter) instead of regular butter or margarine, and coconut palm sugar instead of white refined sugar will all help modify the pleasure spike. These still taste good—salty, buttery, sweet—but don't have the same extreme effect on your dopamine levels. These are small changes—you don't give anything up—but they result in big effects when you are able to back your way out of addiction and into a state of balance, in which your brain and body "crave" healthier choices. Again, no willpower required.

When this downregulation happens, the foods you always crave will become less powerful. You will crave them less and with less intensity as your body shifts from an allostatic state back to a homeostatic one. When you eat, you will still get a pleasure response, but it won't be as extreme, and you will begin to eat less of that thing you thought you had to binge on. This will eventually allow you to eat things that are high in sugar and/or fat without immediately slipping back into an addiction response. You won't have to live in a bubble, constantly terrified that one bite of sugar or carbs or fat will send you into a binge, because you won't be trapped in the stress-response reaction anymore. You will have broken your addiction. As long as you don't revert to overstimulating your pleasure response, you can enjoy these things in moderation and will get a lot more enjoyment out of their natural forms, such as fruit, whole grains, and plant fats. In other words, you'll be able to eat in a way that you used to perceive as impossible. It will feel normal, not out of your control.

The Prime Normalizes Dopamine Centers

We will also normalize the dopamine centers. If you have lost dopamine receptors, you are not getting the same pleasure response you got before. At the same time we will give you other coping mechanisms that will help you not need as much of a pleasure response. I will give you easy strategies to calm your body in other ways. When you reduce emotional pain, you won't feel as strong a need to dull that pain with food.

One of these techniques, which I will talk about in more detail later, is meditation. From a biochemical standpoint, meditation makes a huge difference in how the body handles stress and how the brain responds to stress. I had a patient who began The Prime, and a few weeks in, she told me: "Oh my gosh. I never felt loved by my parents. I was an unwanted birth, and I've carried that with me all this time!" Her body had moved into a state where she was finally able not only to see this but to cope with it and let it go. These things naturally start to unwind as the detoxification process progresses. People begin to understand some of the more deeply rooted things that happened to them in childhood that can make them more susceptible to addiction, and they get to a place where they are finally able to resolve those issues in ways they couldn't before. As the mind and the gut get stronger, you become strong enough to cope with things you may have suppressed.

As you progress through these pages, I'll also tell you more about some specific herbs called *adaptogens* that help normalize the HPA axis and the dopamine pathways. Brahmi helps with the dopamine pathways, while ashwagandha (as I've already mentioned) helps normalize the HPA axis. Yet another technique: keep a cravings journal. When you have a craving, take a few minutes and write down where you think it's coming from. This often results in some pretty major surprises for my patients. In the beginning it may be hard. You may think, "All I want to do is eat this cookie. I don't know why." When you slow it down, asking yourself on a regular basis where the craving is coming from, usually the underlying psychological influences will rise to the surface. You'll learn what's really triggering your HPA axis and what you are trying to escape from with food. This always amazes me.

Sometimes my patients tell me they discover that things they felt they had already dealt with are still simmering under the surface. The point of this exercise is to move the psychological influences from the unknown, subconscious regions of your mind into the known conscious regions of your mind, giving you more control. It is just one more effective tool. Now when you reach for that cookie or soda, you will know: *I want this because I'm lonely. I want this because I'm angry. I want this because I'm filled with grief.* Knowing why can make a big difference in how you choose to respond. With the dietary and other supports you will get from The Prime, the healthier response may finally seem doable to you.

The Prime Recalibrates the Microbiome

Finally, we will change the composition of your gut bacteria, which directly influences cravings and how well the gut works. We will do this by restoring a digestive tract paralyzed by stress, as well as by making a few easy lifestyle changes that will balance your microbiome in a way that makes cravings easier to manage. This is a significant part of The Prime.

Initially, the dopamine spikes and the HPA axis activation are what trigger the addictive process. What happens with food in particular—more so than with any other substance, which is why it, in my opinion, is the most addictive substance of all—is that food alters your gut flora. Now you have this entire other population inside you that makes up 90 percent of your DNA, and it is thrown out of balance and is asking for those same foods you can't seem to quit. Now you are really hooked—both neurochemically and gastrointestinally. Your brain and gut are conspiring against you. Every dietary addition we use in The Prime not only helps downregulate the stress response and normalize dopamine receptors but also encourages more effective digestion and a more body-friendly micro-biome. (I'll talk a lot more about this in the next chapter.)

We will be coming at the problem from all kinds of angles, all designed to work with your body's natural adaptive responses rather than against them. The one thing we *won't* do is start by telling you to eat less and exercise more. Those things will happen spontaneously, if you need them, when your body is ready to accept them. Using these techniques and many more (all easy, all inexpensive), The Prime nudges your body into a new homeostasis. As the highs come down (and the lows come up), your HPA axis calms down and stops pumping you full of stress hormones. This is where we start to see real change. Once you are controlling neuroadaptation instead of your cravings and food addictions controlling you, you will feel real changes in your body and brain. You will feel more control over your behavior. And the foods you love? Despite what you may feel now, and without any conscious forcing, those are going to shift.

CHAPTER 4

IT'S NOT WHAT YOU EAT, IT'S WHAT YOU DIGEST

Your brain is a critical player in food addiction, but another important force is influencing what you choose to eat. It can potentially interfere with every aspect of your health and can also pave the way for overall health, self-control, and effective lifestyle change. This force is digestion.

Ancient physicians knew what modern doctors are only beginning to fully understand: that one of the most important factors in overall health—including weight issues, chronic disease, and brain dysfunction—is the health of your digestive system. An old Ayurvedic saying goes something like this: "It's not just about what you eat. It's about what you digest." This is an essential concept in Ayurvedic medicine and a critical concept for The Prime.

Digestion influences everything about you. A strong digestive tract extracts nutrients from food, fuels your activities, builds and repairs your body, removes toxins from your body, and energizes your brain. Weak digestion results in the accumulation of toxins, or ama, and tissue inflammation, from brain to toe. Weak digestion is the precursor to every chronic disease. Health begins with digestion, and disease starts with impaired digestion. If you don't Prime your digestion for absorption and the proper and prompt elimination of toxins from the body, you cannot achieve health, not to mention weight loss and a clear head.

Because this is so important, I want you to understand how digestion works, both physically and emotionally, so you can better understand how The Prime is helping your body do what it wants to do naturally. Looking at emotions and digestion may seem strange to you, but it is an ancient and complete way to look at this intimate internal process, so stay with me. The more you learn about ancient views on digestion, the clearer the picture of what happens when food takes its long and interesting journey through your body.

The Digestive Journey

The digestive tract is a fascinating part of the body. It is, in essence, a tube. One opening is the mouth, and the other is the anus. It goes through you, but it is open to the outside, so its mechanisms for exchanging material from the outside world with the internal body is highly regulated and protected. You could take any food (or liquid or a pill or even a small nonfood object, such as a capsule with a camera in it for certain exploratory medical procedures) and drop it into one end of the tube and then catch it (maybe with gloves on?) as it comes out the other end of the tube. The journey may take some time—a lot happens from the beginning to the end of those thirty winding feet of tube—but if all goes as it should, what goes in eventually comes out. It may be in an altered form and it may have some missing or added elements, but it goes in and then it comes back out.

This tube is also similar in many ways from one end to the other. The terrain changes a bit, but not all that much. The tissue in your mouth is much the same as the tissue in other parts of your gastrointestinal tract. It is meant to protect the inside of your body by creating a barrier, to excrete substances to help with digestion, and to absorb nutrients, which is why some medications and vitamins can be administered by placing them under your tongue (sublingually). Let's take a look at each part of the digestive tract. We'll see what it does, and we'll consider the Ayurvedic perspective.

DIGESTION AND GOOD TASTE

Tasting food may seem like it's all about pleasure, but it has a functional influence on how well your digestion works. There is a significant connection between the mouth and the nervous system—both the enteric (gut) and the central (brain) branches. Taste is a strong cue to your brain about what kind of digestive enzymes the gut should secrete. The taste of a food sends signals to the brain that prepare the gut to receive that particular food. For this reason, taking certain herbs in liquid or powder form, so you can taste them, makes them more powerful than taking them in a pill form. For example, the taste of certain spices, like those we use in The Prime, sends a signal to the brain to prep the gut for better digestion.

The Mouth

The digestive tract begins with the mouth. It is the window to your gut, the opening of the tube, and the first place where your body begins to break down food in order to extract nutrition. That's why you have teeth, of course. As you grind your food with your teeth, your mouth releases saliva, which contains enzymes that start the digestion process—mostly enzymes that digest carbohydrates, converting them into sugar. The longer you chew, the better the effect, and the easier time you will have digesting carbohydrates. Your mouth also contains a lot of bacteria that secrete not only enzymes but odors and waste. Bacteria live under your gums, and just as in your intestines, you can have a population of bacteria that are doing good things for you, or not-so-good things, such as smelling bad (when your breath smells like sulfur, or something worse) and increasing inflammation (both in your gums and in your body).

The mouth also contains a particularly useful barometer of your digestive health: your tongue. The condition of your tongue, especially first thing in the morning, says a lot about the quality of your digestion because your body excretes waste through the tongue. Do you have a thick white coating? A gray coating? A greenish coating?

Or is your tongue purely pink? In Ayurvedic medicine, a chronic coating on the tongue signals the presence of toxins in your system. Different kinds of coating, coloring, and indentations on the tongue also signal different kinds of digestive and health issues.

WHAT'S THE PH OF YOUR SPIT?

The pH of your saliva can also be an indicator of your digestive and general health. A neutral saliva pH is between 6.8 and 7.0, but if it gets lower than that, your saliva is too acidic, suggesting inflammation (a higher pH means your saliva is more alkaline, which is generally more desirable than saliva that is too acidic). Before you start The Prime, you could test your saliva to see what it is, then track how it changes as you progress through the program. (You can buy inexpensive pH test strips from any pharmacy.) Measure your saliva pH for a few days before you begin the program, so you have a baseline measurement. Just spit into a spoon and place the pH test strip into the sample of your spit. (Don't put the strip in your mouth—there are chemicals on it that I don't recommend ingesting.) Wait two hours after consuming food or drink to test your saliva pH as these can affect your results.

When you begin The Prime, your body will naturally start shedding toxins, which will increase the acidity of your saliva. Because of this, you will probably notice a decrease in your saliva pH as you detoxify, if you are keeping track. This is normal and a sign that The Prime is working. By the end of The Prime, the pH of your saliva will likely be less acidic than when you started, indicating an overall decrease in acidity and toxic load on your body.

The Stomach

After you chew your food and swallow it, it moves quickly through the esophagus with the help of muscles that push the food downward into your stomach. Although the stomach contains digestive enzymes, much of what happens here is mechanical. This is where your food gets mixed—tossed and turned with stomach acid until it gets broken down into more of a slurry than actual chunks of food. (The more you chewed your food, the less work your stomach has to do.) The stomach is the source of most of the mechanical mixing in your digestive process because it is a pouch and has the most room. This is why Ayurvedic physicians recommend that you never eat until you are completely full. Stop when you are 80 to 85 percent full to leave enough space in your stomach for the mixing process.

The stomach is an important organ in Ayurveda. It is connected to the emotions. When you feel sad or emotional, your stomach will have a harder time digesting your food. If your emotions are "undigested" (unrecognized or unprocessed), your food may not get digested well, either. I see this often with children who have unresolved emotions that often manifest as stomach problems. Kids often complain of stomachaches when they aren't feeling well emotionally. Stress signals from the brain can cause nausea, indigestion, stomach cramps, and even actual ulcers in the stomach lining.[1] In Ayurvedic medicine, emotional stress in particular (as opposed to mental or physical stress) is most likely to cause stomach issues, and stomach issues in particular can cause emotional distress. The connection runs both ways.

The Small Intestine

After your stomach has processed your food, it is pushed down into the small intestine, where enzymes secreted by the intestinal lining further digest it. This is also where the food is mixed with more enzymes made by the pancreas that help you break down carbohydrates, fats, and proteins. The small intestine is lined with tiny hairs called *microvilli* that provide a huge surface area for the absorption of usable nutrients extracted from food by the digestive enzymes. These microvilli are embedded in the lining of the small intestine, which is somewhat similar to a fine, tightly woven mesh that should be sound enough to keep toxins and food particles inside the digestive tract while letting only fully digested micronutrients into the bloodstream. This section of the intestine also contains a small amount of intestinal bacteria, but not as much as the large intestine.

The small intestine is extremely important in digestion because this is where most of the nutrition from food is absorbed, or "burned" for fuel. In Ayurveda, this is considered a heat center, or the center for *agni*, the digestive fire. It is no coincidence that the small intestine is susceptible to chronic inflammation, a condition of too much heat.

Agni is an important concept in Ayurvedic medicine because it is the energy of metabolism, turning food into fuel for living, but it also is the digestive fire for emotions, experiences, and everything else we "ingest," physically, mentally, and emotionally. Strong agni signifies a strong digestion. Weak agni creates a backup and increased accumulation of ama, or toxins. Strong agni burns through food and keeps digestion healthy and functioning vigorously, allowing you to absorb nutrients from the food you eat. (Agni is the reason why cold food is generally contraindicated in Ayurveda—heat is required for biotransformation.)

When something goes wrong in the small intestine—for example, people with celiac disease have an immune system that attacks it and destroys the microvilli that absorb nutrients—then there will be problems transforming food into nutrition that feeds the body. In the Ayurvedic view, this dysfunction weakens agni and can interfere with the ability to transform or digest events in our lives that impact our identity or self-concept. It can make people feel more "permeable," just like the gut. They may experience a weakening of self-concept, identity, and feelings of personal power. It can cause difficulty accomplishing things and fulfilling goals, or it can cause procrastination based in insecurity and indecision. The person has lost the "fire" of conviction or the "spark" of a strong personality, becoming more vulnerable to and swayed by outside influences.

The Large Intestine (Colon)

If digestion is occurring properly, by the time food reaches the colon from the small intestine, it has been almost completely digested. All the major digestive processes have been completed by this point, and most of the nutrients have been absorbed. There is still absorption of water and a few nutrients, but otherwise, the large intestine's job is to transform the remaining waste into stool and push it out of the body. The large intestine contains most of the bacteria in the digestive tract. These bacteria form the stool, but (as you will learn in the next chapter) they also are quite closely linked with the nervous system. Most of the process of making waste products "inert" depends on the population of good bacteria in your colon.

In Ayurveda, your colon is also where a sense of stability is located. Ideally, you should feel grounded and secure, but when you are feeling ungrounded, these feelings are linked to a problem in the health of your colon and the bacteria that live within it. Whereas stomach upset is linked to emotional upset, colon upset is more related to disorders of the mind. Many psychological and neurological problems in Ayurveda are linked to colon health, and science is only now uncovering the biochemical basis for this. (This is why enemas can be so important in Ayurvedic treatment of neurological conditions.) Although in the past, the link between the colon and the brain has been a difficult concept for people in the Western world to understand (we see the colon down here and the brain up there), recent research into how gut microbes of the large intestine influence or even control our moods and mental state via the vagus nerve are changing this.[2] We are finally discovering that the condition of the gut bacteria in the large intestine affects the neurochemical balance in the brain. The overgrowth of bad bacteria in the colon is particularly harmful to the blood-brain barrier once the integrity of the matrix of the bowel is impaired.

Peripheral Digestive Organs and Systems

Although they are not technically part of the tube that is the digestive system, some organs and systems directly impact how digestion works. The liver and the lymphatic system, both crucial for detoxification, work side by side with the digestive tract to keep you absorbing nutrients and eliminating waste, while the pancreas is responsible for producing key digestive enzymes that help you digest and extract nutrients from food.

The Liver

One of the liver's most important functions is to screen everything you eat, drink, and ingest for toxic material. When it finds something toxic, it neutralizes the toxin so it can't harm you, by making it water soluble (for excretion through the kidneys) or fat soluble (for elimination through the colon or storage in the body), or if it can't manage the toxin, it binds it to bile and sends it back into the small intestine for another go-around. This is why each time a toxin gets reabsorbed, it gets more toxic. It is getting more concentrated. When toxins overload the liver, they typically are stored in fat cells and/or keep getting sent back through the digestive system, which can cause chronic inflammation in the mucosa that lines the entire digestive tract, eventually damaging it.

But that's not all your liver does. It's one of the hardest-working detoxification organs in the body. It has many jobs, including the following:

- Removing harmful toxins from your blood
- Metabolizing cholesterol
- Fighting infection
- Helping to digest fat via the formation of bile, which the liver secretes into the gallbladder and then into the small intestine

- Storing nutrients and vitamins
- Storing energy in the form of glycogen

In Ayurvedic medicine, the liver isn't just a chemical detoxifier. It is also an emotional detoxifier, helping to break down damaging emotions. Doctors often see people with liver disease who also experience depression, and especially anger and frustration. In earlier times, anger was referred to as bile, which is the substance the liver secretes for removal of waste from the body. This always reminds me of the stereotype of the angry or emotionally volatile alcoholic, which makes sense from an Ayurvedic perspective because alcohol is a strong liver toxin (hepatotoxin) that impedes the liver's ability to break down chemical as well as emotional toxins. You become filled with "bile," and anger turned inward, "unmetabolized," often turns into depression.

Many of my patients with liver problems are in severe stages of depression, and when they begin The Prime, they suddenly go from feeling depressed to feeling angry. They can't understand why—they are typically surprised. Where is all this anger coming from? To me, however, it's perfectly logical. Because the liver's metabolism is beginning to improve, it is working through not only the physical toxins that have built up but the heavy emotional toxins that had piled into such a heap that they were creating depression. Alleviating these, bit by bit, lightens the load, and what was once anger undigested (i.e., depression) reverts back to anger as it clears out of the body. This is fascinating to me because many of these people have spent a lifetime holding on to their anger (and aggravating their livers). They aren't used to being able to release that anger, so when it starts happening spontaneously, they aren't sure what to make of it. Often, they begin to have vivid, sometimes violent dreams, as their brains attempt to process the anger being released from the body. This is a way for the subconscious mind to help "digest" all the anger.

The Pancreas

The pancreas is an integral component in the digestive process. You may think of the pancreas as the organ that makes insulin. One part of the pancreas does this job and is largely responsible for controlling blood sugar levels in the body (because insulin moves sugar from the blood into the cells). The pancreas also makes glucagon, which triggers the liver to break down stored sugar and release it into the bloodstream when needed. Insulin and glucagon work together in a finely tuned balance to keep your blood sugar stable.

But another part of the pancreas also has an important job related to digestion. It makes three major enzymes that are involved in breaking down your food: amylase to break down carbohydrates, lipase to break down fats, and protease to break down proteins. If the pancreas isn't releasing the enzymes that break down your foods properly, then more stress and strain will be placed on the colon to deal with the undigested food. This can cause a lot of digestive issues. For instance:

- If you have an amylase deficiency, more undigested carbohydrates make it to your colon, causing gas and flatulence, but without any bad smell.

- If you have a lipase deficiency, your bowel movements can become oily.

- If you have a protease deficiency, then more proteins make it to the colon, causing gas and flatulence that tends to be pretty stinky.

Keep your pancreas functioning properly and your digestion as well as your blood sugar and insulin levels will remain more stable and functional.

CYTOCHROME P450 ENZYMES: DETOX CENTRAL

A crucial system works in your liver to process toxins. This system consists of enzymes called *cytochrome P450 enzymes*, and they are critical for the metabolism of substances that contain toxins, such as medications, drugs, alcohol, and other chemicals. When I was in medical school, I thought the cytochrome P450 enzymes were so boring because we had to memorize which drugs were broken down through that pathway and which drugs were broken down in other ways. It was just a matter of rote memorization. What I didn't realize was how incredible this system is. It breaks down medications, but it also breaks down environmental toxins, alcohol, recreational drugs, and the toxic by-products of foods, not to mention the toxic by-products of your own metabolism. Through biotransformation, these enzymes convert the toxic by-products into water-soluble or fat-soluble forms so they can be safely eliminated or stored.

The problem is that the more toxins you are exposed to, the more those toxins are competing for the limited spaces the cytochrome P450 enzymes have available. Imagine a really good car wash known for getting cars squeaky clean. This car wash has four bays. If you have four cars at a time that need to be washed, then everything will keep moving, but if twelve cars show up at once, or twenty-four cars, or fifty cars, then that car wash is going to get pretty backed up while each car waits for its turn. Some customers won't wait—they will go back out to the road in a dirty car, or hope it rains, or maybe try to wash their own car at home, but none of those other methods are quite as effective.

Cytochrome P450 enzymes are like that car wash, and if you overload them, you're going to get a backup. If you don't want to get a backup, there are two things you can do:

- Provide a good support staff for the car wash—that is, provide nutrients to nourish and improve the action of these enzymes. The nutrients that support its pathways act as cofactors, boosting the function of the system. They are like the employees at the car wash who keep the place running, take your money, maintain the machinery, and build more bays to manage a higher load. Without the staff, the car wash would break down, and without nutrients, your detoxification pathways wouldn't work either. This is why you will flood your body with nutrients in The Prime and take guggul. Guggul upregulates the expression of these detoxification enzymes, kick-starting your liver into serious detox mode. But we do this only after your liver is fully nourished by the Prime Juice and Prime Broth. Without that nourishment, detox symptoms will be more severe.

- Reduce the number of cars coming in for a wash—that is, reduce your toxin load. Fortunately, The Prime will help you do this easily because of the way it increases your sensitivity to substances that contribute to this toxic load. In fact, many of my patients tell me that after they have been on The Prime for a while, they spontaneously give up smoking, drinking, or recreational drugs. They say things like, "I don't know why, but I just suddenly quit smoking." That's the detoxification power of The Prime.

The Lymphatic System

The lymphatic system is a network of nodes and vessels and valves that lie just under the skin and transport lymph—a clear fluid containing white blood cells and waste products—throughout the body. Lymph is one important method of body detoxification—it helps remove fluid from between cells and keeps white blood cells circulating to fight infection. It also extracts the waste products from your digestive tract, including fat-soluble toxins, and transports them to the lymph nodes. The lymph nodes are concentrated immune cells that destroy harmful agents such as viruses and bacteria and eliminate waste by shuttling it into the bloodstream and out through the kidney and liver.

It's a fairly complex system, but to simplify, I like to think of the lymphatic system as a garbage truck that pulls junk away from your organs and the spaces between your cells and into the lymphatic channels, or highways, so your cells aren't bombarded by waste. This waste moves out through the lymph nodes and then gets channeled through the kidneys and into the bladder for removal from the body or into your venous system, where it is filtered by the liver.

WHAT DOES LYMPH HAVE TO DO WITH DIGESTION?

Conventional medicine views the lymphatic system as part of the immune system, but two thirds of your immune system is located in your digestive tract, both in the form of actual lymph tissue located in the gut, called GALT (gut-associated lymphoid tissue), and in the form of gut bacteria that interact with that tissue. The lymphatic system is also traditionally considered to be part of the circulatory system, even though it does not connect to the heart and is not pumped by the heart. It's more accurate, in my opinion, to classify the lymphatic system as a waste removal system; this is why I chose to discuss it in this chapter, because waste removal is one of the key roles of the digestive system.

Because it is a bit of a lone-wolf system, not pumped by the heart or moved automatically through smooth muscle action as in the digestive tract, lymph easily becomes sluggish and backed up. If this happens, it can't relieve the digestive system of some of its toxic load, which can cause digestion to back up too, as your body becomes less and less able to remove waste from your GI tract. Sluggish lymph also builds up as fluid accumulation throughout your body, making you puffy and chubby looking, although not from fat. You may think it's from fat, which is why I call lymphatic backup Fake Fat.

The reason lymph needs so much help is that it has to move upward, against gravity, without any dedicated internal mechanism pushing it in that direction. The lymph has to make it to the lymph nodes so the toxins in it can get filtered by the immune cells, yet nothing pushes the lymph up except movement, so it can get stuck and pool in the lower body. This is why some people have swollen feet and ankles, especially when they are too sedentary. Some people (like me) are born with fewer lymph nodes and have even more problems with excessive water and lymph accumulation when the body gets inflamed.

The only way to get lymph moving is by moving it manually. You can do this by exercising or just moving around vigorously—muscle action peripherally puts pressure on the lymphatic system's fine network of vessels. The most effective kind of exercises for getting lymph moving are jumping rope and jumping on a trampoline (recently rebranded as *rebounding*)—or just jumping on the ground (although a trampoline makes jumping a little lower-impact). My favorite strategy for getting lymph moving is lymphatic massage, which you can have a professional do, or you can do it yourself. If lymphatic backup and Fake Fat are problems for you, I highly recommend you do a lymphatic massage on yourself daily (I'll tell you exactly how to do it in Chapter 6).

You can change your natural tendency to bloat and swell by changing how efficiently your lymphatic system is working. Several aspects of The Prime directly work on the lymphatics, including lymphatic massage and plant products such as manjistha and guggul.

Do You Have Fake Fat?

Because so many people are prone to lymphatic backup, I want to take a minute to go into a little more detail about this problem, which I call Fake Fat. Many people who believe they have excess fat don't have as much of it as they think they do. Lymphatic backup looks and feels like fat (it is very soft, like a water balloon), but it fluctuates from morning to evening or throughout the menstrual cycle. If you are one of those people who can gain five pounds overnight (or lose five pounds in a week), you are probably plagued with Fake Fat.

Do you have Fake Fat? Let's find out right now. Then, as we get into the details of the program, I will have some special information for those of you with this lymphatic backup. Answer the questions below to determine if this is you.

Is Your Fat Real?

1. Does your weight often fluctuate more than four or five pounds over the course of twenty-four hours?
2. Do you have difficulty sweating, even when you are exercising?
3. Do your rings get stuck by the end of the day because your fingers get puffy?
4. Do you get lines around your ankles where your socks were, or marks from your shoes?
5. Do you have aching in your joints? Do you often feel stiff, especially if you have been sitting for a while?
6. Do you have excessive cellulite? Everybody has some, but do you have large amounts and lots of lumps?

7. For women, do you gain more than five pounds around your menstrual cycle?

If you answered yes to two or more of these questions, then you probably have Fake Fat and should add the optional manjistha powder to your tea in Stage One of The Prime. This will boost your body's efforts to move lymph and reduce Fake Fat more efficiently.

IF YOU HAVE HAD LYMPH NODES REMOVED

People who have had lymph nodes removed, often during cancer treatment (especially breast cancer), have a special problem with lymphatic backup. Swelling, such as in the arm when lymph nodes in the armpit have been removed, can get quite severe, a dangerous condition called lymphedema. If you have had lymph nodes removed, it is especially important for you to practice daily lymphatic massage. You should also add manjistha powder to the tea you will begin drinking in Stage One of The Prime. Manjistha powder comes from the root of the common madder or Indian madder plant, in the coffee family, and it is a powerful lymphatic stimulator. Also, you may want to consider regular professional lymphatic massages. This painless and enjoyable bodywork should be performed by a massage therapist with special training in lymphatic massage. Your doctor should be able to recommend someone, as many of these trained massage therapists work in hospitals and specialize in treating people who have had lymph node surgery. Even if you do get professional lymphatic massages, however, don't underestimate the power of daily self-massage.

When Digestion Goes Wrong

Your body's digestive system should work well enough to absorb the nutrients required by the body to maintain its daily activities and eliminate an average amount of waste and toxins from the external and internal environments. There are many ways that things can go wrong in the digestive tract, however. For example:

- The toxic load can become too high for the body to handle (which is more and more common as our food becomes more processed and our environment becomes more polluted). As the toxins make their way into the digestive tract, they can cause the mucosal lining of the gut to become compromised and inflamed.

- The gut bacteria that make us healthy can become replaced by gut bacteria that compromise health. Also, bacterial overgrowth can release an endotoxin called LPS (lipopoly-saccharides). This toxin is pro-inflammatory, further damaging the gut lining. It has been associated not only with gut dysfunction but also with brain dysfunction, including depression, schizophrenia, and, in research currently being conducted but not yet released, Parkinson's disease.[3] The only way to get rid of LPS is to heal the inflammation in the gut and bring balance back to the normal gut flora ratios.

- Damage to the mucosal lining can cause problems with nutrient absorption, so the body can't process the food consumed. This results in the formation of ama. The organs of detoxification (such as the liver) become overburdened and undernourished. A compromised mucosal lining can also allow food particles to escape from the digestive tract into the bloodstream and overstimulate the immune system (sometimes called "leaky gut syndrome").

Any of these issues could result in leaky gut, constipation, lymphatic backup, liver dysfunction, or insulin resistance. This can trigger inflammation throughout the entire body, resulting in weight gain, brain fog, fatigue, and chronic disease.

How The Prime Specifically Heals Digestion and Optimizes Detoxification

Almost every aspect of The Prime has a positive and therapeutic influence on digestion:

- **Reverses inflammation.** The spices in your Prime Tea and Prime Curry Powder are particularly good at healing inflammation in the gut—especially turmeric, cumin, coriander, fennel, and amla. The curry powder has a strong antioxidant effect, blocking the destructive effects of free radicals and minimizing oxidative stress. The spices also rev up your agni, making your digestive system more efficient at burning off ama within the gut.

- **Repairs leaky gut.** Prime Broth is also a known gut healer because of the glutamine it contains. It is frequently prescribed for healing leaky gut. Triphala also helps repair the gut mucosa.

- **Cleans the blood.** Guggul is particularly good at clearing the macromolecules that have escaped into the bloodstream, so your body's mistaken immune reaction can settle down again. Guggul does this in part by enhancing liver function, which speeds up your body's natural detoxification mechanisms.

- **Rebalances gut bacteria.** The fiber you will begin taking is excellent food for good bacteria, which will help them edge out excess bad guys.

LEAKY GUT SYNDROME

Leaky gut syndrome is a controversial diagnosis. At first, doctors tended to dismiss it as a myth, but now there is a lot of scientific evidence to support its existence. Today, doctors usually admit that it seems to be a real thing, even if they don't totally understand it.[4] Here's what makes sense to me, based on my patients' experiences, medical testing, and research: Leaky gut syndrome happens when the tightly woven mesh in the small intestine, which holds the microvilli that absorb nutrients from food, gets injured and becomes compromised as a filter. This can happen when the small intestine is damaged through inflammation and toxic exposure. It may happen as a consequence of certain medications, such as nonsteroidal anti-inflammatory drugs (NSAIDs), aspirin, immunosuppressants, chemotherapy drugs, or medical procedures such as radiation therapy. It can also be the result of chronic exposure to toxic foods that cause inflammation in the gut. This damage can start long before you ever have any symptoms, and long before you develop any diagnosable chronic diseases.

A protein called zonulin is responsible for moderating the tight junctions in the intestinal mesh, but in some genetically susceptible people, the zonulin pathways become deregulated and the mesh can develop leaks.[5] I believe it is most commonly the result of low-grade chronic inflammation in the lining of the small intestine due to a number of dietary factors (gluten sensitivity, overconsumption of sugar) and environmental factors (food preservatives/additives), which causes ongoing injury to the tissue, eventually resulting in small tears in the mesh.

Whatever the reason the gut becomes leaky, the problem is that things the digestive tract should keep inside escape into the bloodstream. These include not just toxins but food particles that are perfectly harmless within the GI tract but dangerous in the bloodstream.[6] Many food particles, such as proteins, resemble tissues in our own body. For example, gluten resembles thyroid cells. When gluten escapes the digestive tract through a leaky gut, the body perceives an invader and begins to attack the gluten proteins, *and also* the thyroid cells that resemble the gluten proteins. This may be why there seems to be a link between gluten intolerance and thyroid-focused autoimmune diseases such as Hashimoto's and Graves' disease,[7] as well as with other autoimmune conditions.[8] We have seen a big rise in autoimmune diseases in the past few years,[9] especially in women, possibly because many environmental toxins act and look similar to estrogen, and women have more estrogen receptors. Fortunately some tests are being developed that will help us detect this process before it develops into a full-blown autoimmune disease.[10]

In the meantime, repairing a leaky gut can go a long way toward repairing the autoimmune dysfunction in the body. However, once autoimmunity is established, it can take some time to reverse it. It can take the body three to six months to heal a leaky gut, but the clock starts only *when the inflammation and injuring agent is completely removed.* First, we have to calm down the digestive tract, cool the inflammation, and get everything moving along properly again, so the total time to heal can be as long as one to two years.

- **Increases the rate of toxin removal.** The Prime Tea helps remove toxins from the GI tract and moves water-soluble toxins out of the kidneys. Psyllium husks and flax seeds help bind toxins in the GI tract, including environmental toxins such as heavy metals in addition to undigested food and other waste by-products. Guggul also increases the expression of the liver enzymes responsible for detoxification, increasing the efficiency of the liver detoxification pathways. Guggul is also good at breaking down fat and helping to release fat-soluble toxins.

- **Increases detoxification through the lymphatic system and skin.** Dry-brushing with silk gloves (lymphatic massage) moves toxins stored in the lymphatic system into the venous system for the liver to break down (Fake Fat). The Prime Tea and guggul also help flush out the lymphatic system.

- **Nourishes the organs of detoxification.** Because detox pathways in the body are nutrient-dependent and energy-dependent, the Prime Broth and Prime Juice will keep these supplied with what they need to work at capacity. These nutrient-rich additions will also help minimize detox symptoms, which can be caused by insufficient nutrition and insufficient energy from food.

- **Calms the brain.** Your gut and brain are closely linked. Ashwagandha and Brahmi both work on different aspects of the brain, balancing the stress response and reducing cravings, so you can feel less anxious and more focused on how your body feels as it heals. They also help heal the enteric nervous system (the nervous system in your gut).

- **Processes the emotions.** Meditation helps "digest" unprocessed mental and emotional ama, which can sabotage even the best detox programs.

To reiterate the Ayurvedic adage: It's not just what you eat. It's what you digest. I cannot overstate the importance of strong digestion for health and for maximizing the systems of detoxification in the body. Everything begins in the gut, including healing, and we will concentrate on this all-important center, to get your health, your body, and your brain back into Prime condition.

CHAPTER 5

LEAKY BRAIN: UNDERSTANDING THE BRAIN-GUT CONNECTION

Now that we've talked about the brain and the gut, it's time to put them together. The connection between the gut and the brain is truly mind-boggling (or gut-boggling). When I explain the concepts in this chapter to my patients, it often astounds them and is quite frequently the impetus for them to start changing their habits and their thinking about food and their bodies. When you realize how truly integrated your entire system is, and that the main axis of consciousness as well as health runs back and forth between the gut and the brain like a superhighway, you will see your body in an entirely new way—a way that opens the doorway to real change that you can effect on your own.

Let's begin by looking at the brain—but not the brain inside your skull. Let's look at the second brain that lives inside your gut.

The Brain Inside Your Gut

The gut has a mind of its own, and it is called the *enteric nervous system* (*ENS*). The ENS is a network of neurons, neurotransmitters, proteins, and support cells called ganglia, like those found in the brain. The ENS is located just underneath the mucosal lining of the gut, called the submucosa, and also within the smooth muscle tissue of the digestive tract. It's all stretched out along this tube, so it's like a long skinny brain instead of a dense roundish brain, like the one in your skull.

The ENS has about the same number of nerve cells as the entire spinal cord (200 million to 600 million neurons), and just like the brain, the gut sends and receives nerve impulses, records experiences, and responds to emotions. Its nerve cells secrete and are influenced by the same neurotransmitters found in the brain. People don't think of the gut as having intelligence, but it does. Neurons in the gut send signals to the brain for interpretation via the vagus nerve, a long nerve that runs between the brain stem and down through the length of the digestive tract. The brain translates those signals into sensations, thoughts, or emotions. The ENS and the brain communicate all the time. Yet it is not a one-way conversation. We used to believe that the ENS was a kind of servant to the brain, doing what the brain asks, but now we know that the brain is doing most of the listening and the ENS is doing 90 percent of the talking. The gut advises the brain about what to do based on its own condition.

We also used to believe that the ENS relied on the brain operationally, but now we know that this isn't true, either. The ENS is autonomous. Although it communicates with the brain, it does not depend on the brain to work. Even when the vagus nerve is severed, the ENS can still continue to function. It won't function optimally without input from the brain, but it won't die, either. Your ENS not only acts independently, but it can learn and remember; you can teach your gut behaviors (on purpose or inadvertently), such as associating a certain meal with stress (and indigestion) or craving a certain food at a certain time of day.

The ENS has other jobs as well. It controls the muscle action of the GI tract (this wavelike muscle movement is called *peristalsis*, and it keeps everything moving through the system). It also controls the secretion of digestive enzymes that help break down your food and assimilate nutrients from food. Damage to the ENS can hinder enzyme secretion, which can severely impact your body's ability to extract nutrition from food. Enzyme supplements may help a little, but they can never replicate the quality and number of digestive enzymes naturally produced in your own body. Better to repair the ENS.

What fascinates me the most as a neurologist is the way dysfunction in the gut influences dysfunction in the brain, and vice versa. Digestive problems, gut inflammation, leaky gut, and gut flora composition can impact brain health and function, while neuroadaptation, emotional upheaval, and stress can alter digestion, gut flora balance, and the effectiveness of the body's natural systems for detoxification. Here are some other important ways these two systems are connected:

- Nervous system tissue in the gut along with gut bacteria produces 95 percent of the serotonin in your body, and just as much dopamine as your brain produces.[1] These chemicals have a profound influence on your mood and even your personality.

- There are 200 million to 600 million neurons in your gastrointestinal tract, and 90 percent of the signals from the ENS are going from the gut to the brain rather than the other way around, via the vagus nerve. That means what you think and how you feel is impacted by the health and proper function of your gut and digestive processes.

- Recent research has demonstrated that stimulation of the vagus nerve, which connects the gut and the brain, can effectively treat nonresponsive chronic depression.[2] This suggests that depression could be caused or exacerbated, at least in some cases, by a sluggish or dysfunctional gut-brain communication system.

- Bacteria in the gut has a direct effect on the brain, and research suggests that bacteria could control behavior, personality, cravings,[3] food preferences, and disease processes.

Current research is exploring this link and the many ways in which gut bacteria may influence us.

- Many diseases are often foreshadowed by gut health issues. For example, irritable bowel syndrome, constipation, and other chronic digestive issues are often known to occur in patients who later manifest diseases such as multiple sclerosis, Parkinson's, and a range of psychiatric conditions.[4] Research is continuing to unravel this link. For example, Heiko Braak at the University of Frankfurt, Germany, found that Lewy bodies (the protein clumps in the brains of people with Parkinson's) also existed in the gut, in patients who died of Parkinson's disease.[5] Braak theorized that Parkinson's begins in the gut, as the result of an environmental trigger such as a virus, then spreads to the brain.[6] Similarly, the plaques and tangles found in the brains of people with Alzheimer's are also present in their enteric nervous systems. Almost all of my patients with Parkinson's and Alzheimer's disease say that they experienced digestive problems for decades before the onset of their disease, and in general most patients with Parkinson's, Alzheimer's, and multiple sclerosis report problems with constipation. It is common for these patients to be on some kind of laxative or stool softener.

- People with irritable bowel syndrome tend to experience anxiety and depression at a higher rate than others, and people with autism are known to be more likely to have abnormal levels of unhealthy gut bacteria.[7]

- What we put into the gut has a profound effect on mood. This is another interesting area of new research. One recent study showed the effect on brain scans of fat delivered directly into the gut when subjects were shown pictures and exposed to music designed to make them feel sad. Those with the fatty acid injections had a less dramatic sadness response than those who were injected with saline.[8]

- There is also quite a lot of evidence connecting digestive issues such as nausea, abdominal pain, diarrhea, and other GI symptoms to migraine headaches, with digestive symptoms frequently occurring between migraine attacks.

The gut is sometimes called the second brain, but in my opinion, they are both part of the *same brain*. In fact, the tissue in a fetus that becomes the enteric nervous system and the tissue that becomes the brain have the same origin—they both develop from neural crest cells. They really should not be considered separate systems.

How Leaky Gut Leads to Leaky Brain

Now this next part is a little tricky, but bear with me, especially if you really want to understand the science behind why something as seemingly harmless as indigestion can eventually lead to serious brain dysfunction. As a neurologist, I drool over this stuff—it fascinates me, but it is a little technical. I'll do my best to make it clear and straightforward—it all has to do with your body's natural systems for protecting both the brain in your head and the brain in your gut. I want you to understand how these protective mechanisms work, and where they are naturally vulnerable.

You may have heard of the *blood-brain barrier* (let's call it the *BBB*). This is the barrier that keeps the harmful junk floating around in your body out of your central nervous system (CNS), where it could do real damage. The BBB is predominantly located in the brain and spinal cord (your CNS), and endothelial cells are the structural basis of the blood-brain barrier. These cells are woven together to form a physical barrier along the channels leading to the brain and spinal cord, so that these structures are relatively impenetrable and impermeable to proteins and non-lipid-soluble molecules. This prevents the entry of neurotoxic substances into the brain.

BRAIN CHEMISTRY IN YOUR GUT

The enteric nervous system secretes over thirty neurotransmitters, such as serotonin, dopamine, glutamate, norepinephrine, and nitric oxide. These are the same chemicals used in the brain to communicate thoughts, ideas, and moods as well as to store memories. Two neurotransmitters secreted by the ENS that are particularly important and worth talking about here are acetylcholine and norepinephrine.

- **Acetylcholine** in the gut stimulates smooth muscle contractions, increases intestinal secretions, releases hormones, and dilates the blood vessels (you need good blood flow for digestion to occur properly). This is part of the parasympathetic nervous system response in the vagus nerve that tells both the brain and the gut to relax because everything is okay. No worries! Kick back and digest.

- **Norepinephrine** has the opposite effects of acetylcholine. It is part of the sympathetic nervous system response, and gives the brain and gut the "fight or flight" signal when perceiving a danger. This survival response shuts down digestion because the last thing you should be doing when you are in big trouble is wasting valuable energy resources digesting food. Chronic stress, which is a common aspect of modern life, can keep norepinephrine in circulation more often than necessary, chronically hindering digestion.

This isn't a completely impenetrable barrier, however. Some substances need to enter the brain for nourishment and function, such as glucose, amino acids, purine bases, nucleosides, and choline. A few drugs can also penetrate this barrier. Essentially, these substances that the brain needs have a "password" that lets them through the barrier. This password is regulated by the glial cells, which are like the bouncers for the BBB. These glial cells not only hold the endothelial cells together (blocking the doors) but also produce useful anti-inflammatory factors. If these glial cells are injured, however—if somebody takes the bouncer out—then they produce inflammatory molecules that loosen the junctions and allow cracks in the barrier, increasing the permeability of the BBB.[9] This is bad news for the brain, because anything can get in. Examples include irritants that could cause brain inflammation and white blood cells that could attack the structures of the brain and cause lesions, as happens in diseases like multiple sclerosis.

When it's working properly, however, the BBB is quite effective. The good stuff gets in, and the BBB also lets certain things out. Even the brain needs to take out the trash; excess neurotransmitters, hormones, waste products, and other things it needs to get rid of are allowed out the door. Otherwise, the BBB keeps the brain relatively separate from the blood circulating throughout the body.

This is all common knowledge for most doctors. Yet there is more to the story. The brain in your gut, the enteric nervous system, has its own similar mechanism protecting it. This is called the *gut-blood-brain-barrier* (let's call it the *GBBB*). The blood-brain barrier is well studied, but the gut-blood-brain barrier is much less understood. In fact, most neurologists don't even know it exists and therefore don't realize that the things that can disrupt the GBBB are also capable of disrupting the BBB. Most of this information is in gastroenterology journals, which neurologists generally aren't reading, unless they are looking for the gut-brain connection, like I am.

The GBBB is constructed in a similar way to the BBB, with endothelial cells woven around the digestive tract, especially around the parts that include the nerves of the enteric nervous system. Around the ENS, the endothelial cells are woven together much more tightly than in other areas of the digestive tract. Like the capillaries in the central nervous system that lead to the blood-brain barrier, the GBBB also includes glial cells that hold the endothelial cells together, forming tight junctions, sealing the nerves away from the influence of toxins, waste products, and anything else that could damage the ENS. They perform the same type of "bouncer" function.[10]

The problem with the GBBB is that it is more vulnerable to penetration than the BBB, and here's why: Your digestive tract *must allow nutrients out.* Most of the gut must be semipermeable to allow for the necessary diffusion of nutrients to take place between the gut and the blood. It should not allow large food molecules (such as gluten) into the blood, but it is designed to feed the body with nutrients from the food you eat. That means the GBBB must simultaneously guard the nervous system tissue and let nutrients out from all the food you eat to nourish your entire body. This bouncer has to let a lot more guys out the door, without letting anybody in. This involves some tricky multitasking and selective security.

In the GBBB, however, the threat lies within, not without, as it does for the BBB. What you eat and are otherwise exposed to (such as drugs, medications, or chemicals) is already inside the digestive tract. The bouncers can't do anything about what you put in your mouth. This makes the GBBB more vulnerable from the inside. When the gut is exposed to continuous toxins and "new to nature" compounds such as chemical preservatives, food dyes, overly processed foods, sodas, and inflammatory foods such as gluten and refined sugars, the gut mucosa becomes chronically inflamed and the tight junctions of the GBBB loosen up and become permeable all along the gut, and they can no longer protect the ENS.

Now you've got a problem because when the gut mucosa becomes too permeable, not only does it allow large, undigested particles to escape into the bloodstream, which stimulates an overreaction of the immune system, but it also allows toxins such as LPS (lipopolysaccharide, an inflammatory endotoxin that is a by-product of gut bacteria die-off) to enter the submucosal layer, resulting in harm to the glial cells protecting the ENS. When the glial cells are injured, the ENS loses its protection. This subsequently leads to damage of the nerves of the ENS that coordinate all of the processes necessary for normal digestion,[11] and now you've got not just gut permeability but nerve injury and dysfunction. This is essentially "brain damage" to your gut and is as devastating to the gut (and all its processes, including digestion and nutrient absorption) as a spinal cord injury would be to your arms and legs.

Now for the link to the brain: Once you've got a leaky gut and injury to the ENS, the brain in your head is at risk, too. The same inflammatory particles that can break down the GBBB, once they escape the gut and travel to the brain via the bloodstream, can have a similar effect on the blood-brain barrier, breaking it down and eventually entering the brain. You don't want those troublemakers loose in your bloodstream, but once they get in there, they can go anywhere, and they often end up attacking the brain. This is why I often say that leaky gut leads to leaky brain. Once you open the door to the brain, all kinds of dysfunction and degeneration can result.

The bottom line is that gut health mirrors brain health, and gut dysfunction can result in brain dysfunction, and now you understand how. I consider the nerves in the gut the "canary in the coal mine" for the nerves in the brain. What happens to your ENS in your gut can eventually happen to the neurons in your brain. There is just a time lapse. This is why I can take a patient with Parkinson's disease and turn that disease process back in the other direction by focusing on improving digestion. If you don't fix injury in the gut, the brain cannot heal. Fix the gut, stop the brain damage in the gut, and the brain in your skull has a chance at recovery.

WHAT DOES LYMPH HAVE TO
DO WITH THE BRAIN?

Lymphatic vessels are located throughout the body, aiding with immunity and waste removal, but the one place Western science has always believed those valuable vessels *didn't* exist was the brain . . . until now. A recent study that could dramatically alter how neuroscientists understand brain function[12] revealed that researchers have discovered functional lymphatic vessels lining the dural sinuses in the brain. Previously, scientists knew that immune cells existed in the brain but never fully understood how they got there. Now that we know there is indeed a lymphatic system within the central nervous system, we can better understand the brain's own ability to both bring immune cells in and send waste out of the brain.

While this was a big leap forward for Western neuroscience, this is also something Ayurvedic medicine has understood for quite a long time. Specifically, Ayurvedic physicians often explain that many neurological problems are related to the brain's inability to detoxify properly. Before I was trained in Ayurveda, when I often took my patients to see Ayurvedic physicians, about one-third of my MS patients were told their brains were not draining waste properly. I hadn't learned about this yet (no one in Western medicine had), so I couldn't understand what they meant. Now I do. Many of the healing herbs these physicians commonly prescribe for neurological conditions are those that increase lymphatic flow—especially manjistha powder. This makes sense to me now, and doesn't surprise me, either. It's just one more example of how we are just starting to uncover what Ayurveda has known all along.

The Microbiome: Your Partner in Prime

There is one more player in this scenario to consider and it is a pretty major one, playing its own game while you and your central and enteric nervous systems all try to get along. It is a partner to your nervous systems, especially the one in your gut. It is highly influential in almost everything you do, even though it is, essentially, made of little aliens that are not even a real or original part of your body. I'm talking about your microbiome.

The *microbiome* is a community of bacteria that live inside your digestive tract, primarily in your large intestine, or colon. Each one of us has two to three pounds of bacteria there—bacteria that do not come from us and are not technically part of us. The Institute of Functional Medicine likes to say that in one gram of stool, we have more bacteria than there are stars in the known universe.[13] While this may not be technically or mathematically exact, it is surprisingly close and can help us comprehend just how many bacteria we have living inside of us. A lot! And because each one of those bacteria has its own DNA, that is a lot of nonhuman, microbial DNA in our bodies, exerting a constant and persistent influence. Interestingly, these bacteria don't just sit there in our gut gently helping us digest food. They have a huge impact on gut function and, by extension, brain function.

The microbiome (sometimes called *gut flora* or *gut bacteria*) has been all over the scientific news lately because researchers have become enamored with studying it and how pervasive its influence is on almost every part of our health. We now know that the microbiome is quite active in both helpful and intrusive ways. You may have heard about "bad" and "good" gut bacteria. In reality, there are three types of bacteria: "good," "bad," and "neutral," or in more technical and descriptive terms, "symbiotic," "parasitic," and "commensal." What this really means is that certain bacteria, which we call "good bacteria," have evolved to be in a symbiotic relationship with the human body. What is good for them is good for us, and what is good for us is good for them. They help us by producing vitamins, digestive enzymes, hormones, and other compounds that enhance digestion and nutrient absorption, provide support for organ function, and even support brain function.

Other bacteria are neutral—they exist but they aren't particularly helpful or hurtful (as far as we know, currently). They are hanging out and getting a free ride, but it doesn't seem to cost us anything. Finally, there are also bacteria that have not evolved with us. We call these "bad bacteria," and while they are not parasites in the way most medical doctors think of parasites (such as tapeworms or leeches), they fit the definition because they live in us and benefit at our expense. They are opportunistic and what's good for them is bad for us; these bacteria happen to feed on things that are detrimental to our health, such as excessive sugars or fats. They produce toxic by-products from what they eat that harm us and even persuade us (biochemically) to crave and eat more sugar and fat, especially the highly processed kind that they can easily access.

There has been a lot of research recently into the notion that our cravings, weight, and even personality are controlled in part by our gut bacteria. The bad guys who are busy crowding out the good guys have, in the interests of their own survival, figured out how to manipulate the host (that's you) by sending their own signals to the brain: signals like "Eat sugar now!" or "We need French fries!" They can even make you feel rotten until you obey their commands. They do this via neurotransmitters that they produce and send to your brain. They can make you feel depressed, or anxious, or send you serious cravings you think you can't possibly ignore. It sounds like science fiction, but research is bearing this out,[14] and anyone with a food addiction can attest that those cravings seem to overtake their brains. They eat with a feeling that they are not in control of their behavior, and it's true. They are not in control. The gut bacteria are. This is part of the process in which people become neuroadapted and addicted to certain foods—these altered signals coming from the gut contribute to cravings and the feeling of dependence. When your gut bacteria want it, you feel like you need it.

For example, one interesting study has shown that when the gut bacteria of mice are altered through fecal transplants, the mice's behavior changes. Fecal transplants are a cutting-edge area of research. It may sound gross—fecal bacteria are transplanted from one organism to another—but it's a useful way to directly impact gut bacteria composition immediately. Fecal transplants have a dramatic effect on the microbiome, and also on behavior, as this study showed. Mice with more active and exploratory behavior were given fecal bacteria from timid mice, and subsequently they became more timid and less willing to explore their living environment. When timid mice were implanted with fecal bacteria from more adventurous mice, they became braver and more exploratory, no longer hiding in the dark but venturing out into new areas of their enclosures.[15]

Even more fascinating, the brain chemistry of the mice changed after the fecal transplants—adventurous mice had more brain-derived neurotrophic factor (BDNF), whether they were adventurous in the beginning or adventurous after the fecal transplants. Mice that were more timid, either before or after the fecal transplant, had less of this beneficial brain chemical.[16] Clearly, gut bacteria affects brain chemistry, which affects behavior. However, your ENS should be the one in charge of these decisions, with the support of your good gut bacteria, not your bad.

There is also an interesting case study linking body weight to the microbiome composition. In 2015, the Infectious Disease Society of America reported via *Science Daily* that a woman was successfully treated for a dangerous infectious condition called *Clostridium difficile* by receiving a fecal transplant from an overweight donor. The woman had always been of normal weight. The transplant saved her life, but afterward she rapidly gained thirty-five pounds. The change in her microbiome to more closely resemble the microbiome of an overweight person changed her eating behavior and her body weight![17]

I have been consistently surprised by how much even basic personality traits can shift as the gut flora changes. Personality traits we think are uncontrollable, negative traits we think are just part of who we are, are often linked to imbalances in the digestive system. I had a patient who was the CEO of a company. He was in his sixties, and he was a competitive, aggressive person who was having problems with mental focus. When he met me, he reported that part of his problem was that he was (pardon his French) "an asshole."

"Really?" I said. "Well, you may think that's what you are, but maybe it's just an imbalance in your digestion." Obviously being an unpleasant person isn't a disease, but could his behavior be gut-related? I thought so.

Sure enough, after I put him on The Prime, he came into my office one day and said to me, "Oh my God! It turns out I'm not such a bad guy after all. That was just me, out of balance." He still had an intense personality, but he was much less impatient, more focused, more emotionally flexible, and more reasonable.

Keep in mind that there are billions of these bacteria, and each has its own preferences and functions. Ideally, we live with a balance that works for us—mostly good and neutral bacteria with limited numbers of the bad guys, who are kept in check by the good guys. A body system with a high diversity of bacteria tends to do better because any one colony of "bad" bacteria will exert less of an influence. Trouble starts when the bad bacteria get too numerous, which can happen due to lifestyle changes. In just twenty-four hours, your gut population can change dramatically according to what you do, what you eat, and how relaxed or stressed you are. If you feed the bad bacteria what they like (such as refined sugar) and starve the good bacteria by not feeding them what they like (such as fiber), the bad bacteria become too numerous and their effects on you more dramatic. Fortunately, if you can change your gut bacteria unfavorably in twenty-four hours, you can also change them favorably in twenty-four hours.

The microbiome has also evolved to get involved with your digestive processes in useful ways (such as producing enzymes that help with digestion) and detrimental ways. Remember the security breach I told you about, when injured glial cells loosen cell junctions and allow damaging substances into the bloodstream, which can then travel to the brain? One of the harmful effects of certain types of "bad" gut bacteria happens when they die off. Endotoxins that live in the cell walls of these bacteria get released, which can cause inflammation and damage to your glial cells, contributing to leaky gut and, by extension, leaky brain. The fewer of these bad guys that you have, the better, because their presence infects our brains with endotoxins from our guts.

Studies in this area will continue to inform us about this complex, multifunctional brain-gut connection, including my own research—I am working with a group right now to set up a study showing the relationship between the gut and the brain, and specifically how the principles of The Prime can change the clinical course for patients with neurodegenerative conditions. I wanted to pursue this area because so many of my patients come in complaining of trouble focusing or concentrating. They wonder if they have "adult ADHD," or they have anxiety or depression or disruptive premenstrual syndrome (PMS) symptoms. They have brain fog, they have trouble sleeping, or they just don't have any energy. Many of these patients are in their twenties and thirties and complain of dementia symptoms, terrified that they have early-onset Alzheimer's or some other degenerative disease. I look at them thinking, *It's not physiologically possible for you to have dementia—you are too young!* We would have a serious crisis if people in their twenties and thirties were developing dementia—and yet that's what it looks like from their descriptions.

But that's not what it is. Many of these younger patients who already think they have five or six neurological problems (attention deficit/hyperactivity disorder [ADHD], early-onset dementia, depression, anxiety, insomnia), who think they need or may already be on multiple medications, are completely ignoring job one: fixing their digestion. Typically, they have a dysfunctional ENS that has ceded control to opportunistic gut bacteria, and they now have a leaky gut and a leaky brain. They have slipped into a toxic inflammatory state and are quite literally malnourished. Now, even when they eat healthy food, they can't absorb it anymore, and their brains are no longer in touch with what they should and want to eat, so the problem keeps getting worse.

The fact, however, is that the connection is there right now, and proven, and you don't need to wait for medical schools to teach the next generation of neurologists about the gut-brain connection. We know right now that microbial dysfunction in the gut can and usually does eventually result in dysfunction in the brain, unless you intervene before the blood-brain barrier suffers severe injury and loses its integrity.

THE ALZHEIMER'S CURE?

For the first time, a study has demonstrated that personalized and multifaceted lifestyle intervention can reverse memory loss and other symptoms of Alzheimer's and sustain those improvements over time. The study, conducted by Dr. Dale Bredesen at UCLA and the Buck Institute for Research on Aging, used a thirty-six-point therapeutic program involving a broad range of changes, including many of the steps I recommend in The Prime.[18] These included the following:

- Added spices and herbs such as curcumin (extracted from turmeric), ashwagandha, and Brahmi
- Digestive tract repair via increasing the intake of good bacteria
- Reduction of inflammatory foods such as gluten and processed foods
- Meditation
- Increasing sleep hours
- Optimizing oral hygiene
- Moderate exercise
- Fasting twelve hours between dinner and breakfast

This study is significant because it demonstrates the power of relatively simple lifestyle modifications for making a real impact on diseases previously thought to be progressive and incurable.

What Ayurveda Has Known All Along

Nowhere is this connection between the gut and the brain more perfectly understood than in Ayurvedic medicine, which teaches that all health begins in the gut, including brain health. When I started my Ayurvedic training, the first thing I learned was that no treatment for any condition starts before first addressing digestion. In Ayurveda, the term *digestion* encompasses all phases of that process: absorption of nutrients from food, elimination of waste products, and detoxification of residual toxins left from both food and the by-products of metabolism. In Ayurvedic medicine, the force that governs all this is called *agni*. I've already introduced you to this word, but as a reminder, agni is the digestive fire. It is the energy that fuels digestion, burning through food for energy and processing waste. It is located in your small intestine. Remember, we are talking about Ayurveda now, so this is different from how Western medicine perceives the body. You can't see agni on any kind of imaging equipment because it is really just a way of talking about the energy in the body responsible for digestion.

Other kinds of agni in the body also do the work of transformation. They "digest" any experience you have—physical, emotional, spiritual. However, until your primary agni in your gut is strong, these other transformative agnis won't function properly either. In other words, until your digestion is working well, your brain can't properly manage and integrate all the other parts of your life.

This is simple, really. When people improve digestion, have a bowel movement every day, and don't get bloated after meals, it makes a huge difference in how well they start "digesting" experiences, including early memories and traumas. Once digestion, or the primary agni, is fired up and functioning well, the sub-agnis can kick in, processing and working through and finally moving past psychological issues that may have been "stuck" in your body for decades. Just imagine if you ate a meal and it was stuck in your body for twenty to thirty years, and then you finally digested it and got rid of the waste from it. This is how it feels to finally be able to digest and move on from past experiences.

Psychological issues can feel overwhelming—sometimes even more overwhelming than physical issues, especially since they often occur together. The good news is that they are linked, both in their dysfunction and in their solution. When you heal the physical aspects of the body, the psychological aspects tend to follow suit, often resolving themselves with minimal effort. The problems you thought you could never tackle become much easier to process and overcome, and that's a huge relief to a lot of people.

In the same way that healthier lifestyle habits and weight loss become spontaneous on The Prime, this psychological healing also feels spontaneous. Even if it doesn't all resolve itself, The Prime often puts my patients into a mental space where they finally feel ready to tackle a deep-seated issue. They decide they are ready for counseling or some other method of dealing with the problem they have pushed down and ignored for so long. They are more receptive and they are more resilient. You can be, too.

Now you understand why the gut is more than just the second brain. It is *the brain*, intricately and intimately connected with the brain in your head. They are one and the same, each talking to the other, sending messages back and forth, resolving issues and working to keep you in balance—physically, mentally, emotionally, and spiritually. It all begins with healing the gut, and that doesn't take heroic efforts. It's systematic. It's as simple as Priming your body so it can function the way it is meant to function, and all it takes is putting the right things into the system.

PART THREE

The Prime

CHAPTER 6

THE FOUR STAGES

There is no such thing as a one-size-fits-all diet, not to mention a one-size-fits-all detox. Conventional Western medicine tends to isolate a symptom and treat it the same way in every patient, but natural medicine doesn't work like that. We individualize. Every body, every brain, every gut, and every person's biochemistry is unique, not to mention constantly changing. In my clinic, I customize programs for my clients based on their genetic predisposition, health situations, lifestyle tendencies, and symptom profiles. In a book, this is obviously impossible.

But we are making some customizations already. Remember the Fake Fat quiz you took in Chapter 4? That was the first one, and I want to kick off this section of the book with the next method for tailoring the plan to your uniqueness. Now that you know all about how your brain and gut work together, I want to help you determine how smart your gut is right now. This will directly impact how quickly you move through the program. You've probably heard of an IQ test. Maybe you've even taken one. But have you taken a Gut IQ Test?

Your Gut IQ

How smart is the brain in your gut? How functional is your brain-gut connection? How much damage has your enteric nervous system sustained? How easy will it be for you to reverse the dysfunction and start healing? It's time to find out.

Your score will translate into a minimum number of weeks that you should spend at each of the four Prime stages. If you have a smarter gut, you can move through the program quickly. If you have a dumber gut (which is quite common, so don't be surprised or offended if this is you!), you will be much better served by moving through the program more slowly, letting every stage really work in your body and minimizing uncomfortable detox symptoms.

The Gut IQ Test

For each question, think about your life and your symptoms during the past year. Do you have the experience *never, rarely, sometimes, often,* or *always*?

1   I am constipated.   _____

2   I feel bloated, especially after eating.   _____

3   After eating, I get congested or I get phlegm in my throat.   _____

4   After eating, I get heartburn or acid indigestion.   _____

5   I get a lot of gas and flatulence, especially after eating.   _____

6   My tongue is coated with a thick whitish film, especially in the morning.   _____

7   In the morning, I feel foggy and muddled—I don't have a clear head. It takes me a while to feel like I'm really awake.   _____

8   My body feels heavy and slow. _____

9   I feel tired during the afternoon (starting around 2 p.m.), even when I had eight hours of sleep. _____

10   After eating, I feel out of breath. I tend to feel that something is not functioning properly in the body. _____

11   I feel lazy and unmotivated. I can't seem to break out of this feeling of malaise. _____

12   I have congested sinuses or lungs, and/or chronic allergies. _____

13   I feel mentally cloudy most days. I don't have that "sharp mind" I used to have. _____

14   I tend to spit repeatedly or have a bad taste in my mouth. _____

15   Often I have no taste for food and no real appetite. _____

16   I have a dull, heavy, achy feeling in my stomach, like I am carrying a weight around. _____

17   I get colds and other minor viruses frequently. It seems like I catch everything. _____

18   I don't have a bowel movement every day—maybe every other day, or even just once, twice, or three times a week. _____

19   I get out of breath from minor exertion, like walking up a few stairs or walking quickly. I know I'm not that unfit! _____

20   Exercise, or physical exertion in general, exhausts me rather than energizes me. _____

After you've answered all the questions, tally up your score:

Point totals:

Never answers:	_____ × 0 points =		0 points
Rarely answers:	_____ × 1 point =		_____ points
Sometimes answers:	_____ × 2 points =		_____ points
Often answers:	_____ × 3 points =		_____ points
Always answers:	_____ × 4 points =		_____ points
TOTAL SCORE:			_____ **points**

50–80 points: The Gentle Track—four weeks per stage. Your gut definitely needs some work, but don't feel bad; this is quite common. When I was first introduced to Ayurveda, while I suffered from migraine headaches, my score was in this range. Life in our modern world is particularly conducive to gut and brain degradation, and many of my patients fall into this category. I strongly suggest you move through the program slowly. Trust me, going slowly can sometimes be the fastest way to success. Take a good four weeks for each stage—that may seem like a long time, but at this rate, the changes will really stick.

People tend to think that the faster they go, the more effective a program will be, but it's actually the opposite. Fast results could come with uncomfortable detox symptoms that you won't be able to manage, that could compromise your ability to stick with the program. They also often result in a relapse, with subsequent weight gain. People often gain back even more weight than they lost and can find themselves with worse brain fog and lower energy.

Also, for this program, each stage will work best if the previous stage has truly had a chance to do what it is designed to do. For example, until you get the digestion and lymphatic system working better, it won't help to work on cravings. Until you increase your nutritional support, you can't really ask your liver to work harder. Each stage builds on the next.

Trust me when I tell you that there is real wisdom in progressing slowly. Imagine if you tried to build a house as quickly as possible. Just because you really want your house to be built doesn't mean you should rush through with a slapdash foundation. You don't start building the rooms until the foundation is set and strong, and you don't start decorating the rooms until you have the walls and the roof up. You could even take longer than four weeks for each stage, or break the stages down into parts, if that feels more comfortable to you. There is absolutely no hurry. The first time I did this program, I spent two months in each stage. If that sounds fine to you, I encourage this pace. Slow changes become permanent changes, and your body needs time to adjust as it slowly releases toxic materials that impede your progress. The point of this program is to lose the sludge and the weight once, and never gain it back.

20–50 points: The Moderate Track—three weeks per stage. You have an average-intelligence gut, but your gut could definitely be smarter, and it's definitely impacting your brain function and energy level. On The Prime, your detox symptoms won't be as severe as someone who has a higher score, so you can move along a bit faster, if you choose. Of course, you don't have to move faster. You can still take the Gentle Track, and I would even encourage you to do so. Move through each stage at a pace that feels right to you, but you can go as quickly as three weeks per stage, based on your score. No faster, though!

1–20 points: The Fast Track—two weeks per stage. You have a pretty smart gut, and that's good news! You probably aren't far from your health and weight goals, but you still need a little push to get you there. Even smart guts can achieve genius status! Even though you probably feel pretty good, you could be thinking even more clearly, have more energy, and finally get rid of those last few pounds. After The Prime, you'll also be less susceptible to environmental influences that can tip you easily from feeling good to out of balance. You can move through the program pretty quickly. Two weeks at each stage should do the trick, although, again, if you prefer to go more slowly, go ahead! Make it your Prime.

No matter what your score, The Prime will help you turn things around by building a smarter gut. If your gut is "dumb" because it is malfunctioning, it allows gut bacteria to call the shots and run your choices and even your mood via neurotransmitters sent to the brain. The result is that you can't follow a diet. The urge to eat foods that lead to weight gain and disease is simply too strong because it is coming directly from your bad gut bacteria and "passing" as neuronal signals to your brain via the vagus nerve. This is not a war of willpower—this is a biochemical battle.

The answer to losing weight and regaining neurological function is to make the gut smarter by bringing the ENS back online. When this happens, the ENS can override the cravings and other negative effects being initiated by opportunistic gut bacteria. The best way to do that is to fix the digestive system, cultivate a gut environment that allows good bacteria to flourish, improve nutrient absorption, and provide the body with nutrient-dense food so the ENS can heal and start working again. This is a big part of what The Prime accomplishes for you.

When Weight Loss Becomes Spontaneous

As your gut becomes smarter, its communication with your brain can resume and become stronger and clearer. Finally, your conscious mind will begin to remember and understand which foods are toxic. As your ENS begins to reassert its control, your body will respond appropriately when you eat something toxic or harmful by making you feel nauseated or "spacey." Your body will immediately try to flush it out, which could result in vomiting or diarrhea or just stomach pain. You will begin to notice this rejection of certain foods during The Prime, and this is precisely why weight loss won't involve willpower. It will be spontaneous because your body will be rejecting the foods that lead to weight gain.

Foods you once tolerated when your gut was "dumb" and the bad bacteria were in charge will no longer be tolerated, and that's when true dietary change can finally occur: when your gut/brain communication is intact. Once your ENS is in charge again, cravings begin to normalize because your ENS and good gut bacteria work for the benefit of your body, not the benefit of parasitic bacteria. The ENS also becomes more efficient at coordinating the detoxification and digestion process—because it is smarter!

The bottom line is that you don't need more willpower. You need a smarter gut. This is why you can be smart in other areas of your life, such as in your career or personal life, but still not able to change how you eat. It is not a personality flaw. It is a gut bacteria flaw.

Even better news is this: If you thought your brain was smart before, just wait until your gut becomes smart, too. This was my biggest surprise. I always thought I was pretty smart, but once I repaired my digestion, I became smarter and more creative than I ever imagined I could be, and I see the same thing happening with my patients. So many of them launch new careers or get promoted in their current ones after completing The Prime. They start companies. They find better relationships. They thrive. A dysfunctional gut leads to a dysfunctional brain, but a smarter gut leads to a smarter brain and a smarter life.

Now that you know your pace and your Gut IQ, you are ready to begin! You will get the most benefit if you do every part of the program, in the order I have laid out. Each component works together to heal the gut mucosa, restore beneficial gut bacteria, remove toxins, reduce inflammation, reduce cravings for addictive foods, normalize brain function, and improve the absorption of micronutrients from the foods you eat. As you move through the stages, the most important thing you can do is pay attention. Notice how you feel. Notice what your body is doing. Notice how foods taste, and how those tastes slowly begin to change. As best you can, try not to eat out of sheer habit. Notice whether you really want something. If you do, have it. If you suddenly feel a little less interested in eating those things you used to love, pay attention to that and respect it. Your body is changing and becoming more sensitive to the effects of your lifestyle, and it will alert you when you do something it doesn't like.

Finally, I hope you will approach these weeks with a sense of optimism and pleasure. This is not a program of denial or pain. Although you may experience some minor detoxification symptoms, I will help you along the way to minimize any discomfort. The prize at the end of The Prime is a body that responds more quickly to changes, and a mind that is more attracted to a lifestyle geared toward glowing health, high energy, a vigorous constitution, and a normal body weight. Let's get your biochemistry working for you, not against you. Let's jump in and get you Primed!

ACTIVATE A BIOCHEMICAL SHIFT

I n Stage One, we are going to begin to make the colon and the lymphatic system more efficient so they can begin to clear out the ama sludge along the primary detoxification pathways. This is an important first step and a level-one purge of the most superficial layer of ama that is getting in your body's way. To achieve this, you will also open up the pathways through the kidneys, so expect to urinate a little more than usual. You can't flush out the pipes if they are clogged. You will also be moving things along at a faster rate through the colon than they may have been moving before, while nourishing the garden of your gut flora. Don't worry; it's going to feel great!

Remember that you don't have to stop eating any food or start doing any exercise, *unless you feel like it.* If something you were eating before suddenly doesn't seem as appealing or suddenly doesn't agree with you, try skipping it, just to see how you feel.

STAGE ONE SNAPSHOT

Please do the following in the timeframe your Gut IQ Test at the beginning of this chapter indicates:

- **DRY-BRUSH DAILY.** Dry-brush your skin before your daily morning shower using raw silk gloves or an actual brush designed for dry-brushing.

- **SIP PRIME TEA.** Make Prime Tea in the morning and sip it throughout the day. (Recipe to follow.) If you have a particular problem with lymph accumulation (see the Fake Fat quiz, page 88), add 1/2 teaspoon manjistha powder to your tea. If you have excess gas or bloating, add 1/2 teaspoon fenugreek seeds.

- **TAKE TRIPHALA.** Take 1,000 milligrams of triphala every evening before bed with a full glass of room-temperature water (it is easiest to find in capsule form, but you can also mix the powdered form into your water). See Resources for the kind I use and recommend.

- **FLUSH WITH FIBER.** Take fiber every other night, before bed: mix 1 teaspoon each of ground flax seeds and psyllium husks into a glass of room-temperature water and drink. You can take your triphala with your fiber drink.

Now let's look more closely at each element, so you know how and why I am asking you to do it.

Dry-Brushing

Dry-brushing is the process of exfoliating the skin before bathing. It is different from using an exfoliating product with water, such as in the shower. Instead, sans water, you massage the skin with a special brush or glove with a rough surface. (You can easily find dry brushes at most health or natural products stores). In Ayurveda, dry-brushing is called *garshana* and the preferred tool is a raw silk glove. I prefer this, and these gloves are inexpensive and available online. Whichever you use, dry-brushing accomplishes two primary goals:

1. It removes dead layers of skin so the body can more efficiently excrete toxic material. Remember, we are unclogging, and layers of dead skin cells can clog or reduce the efficiency of sweat glands. Dead skin cells are also a type of body waste, and sloughing them off removes this waste.

2. It targets the lymphatic system, which is directly beneath the skin. Dry-brushing is incredibly important for the lymphatic system. You have already learned that your lymphatics don't have a pump. When you move them, they move. Without movement, they have no momentum. Manually massaging the skin toward the heart and in the direction of the lymph nodes gets the lymph moving more vigorously, which increases the body's detoxification rate. Essentially, you are helping to direct the biochemical sewage through the channels and into the lymph nodes, where it can be eliminated. One of the reasons why people develop inflammatory problems in the joints, including arthritis, has to do with lymph accumulation. Cellulite is also a condition exacerbated by backed-up lymphatics. Any place where you have a lot of cellulite should be a particular focus of your lymphatic mas-

sage. Once you get the lymph moving, the fluid content of your fat cells decreases, which reduces the dimpled appearance of cellulite.

I would like you to practice dry-brushing for five to ten minutes every morning before your shower. If you miss a day here and there, don't worry about it. However, you should aim to do a good thorough dry-brushing session at least five or six days a week. Here's how:

Garshana Lymphatic Massage

1. Start with dry, clean skin (since this is before your shower—you don't have to be *squeaky* clean, but you shouldn't have any lotion or oil on your skin).

2. Using silk gloves or a brush, vigorously massage your wrists and the tips of your elbows in circles, then massage with long strokes up from your fingers to the top of your upper arm, directing lymph to the nodes under the arms.

3. Massage your stomach and buttocks in circular motions.

4. Massage your knees in a circular motion, then massage your thighs in long strokes up the leg, directing the lymph to the lymph nodes in the groin area.

5. End with your ankles and feet, massaging them in circles. Then massage up your calf in long strokes using medium to firm pressure.

6. Take your shower.

Prime Tea

This tea is a cornerstone of The Prime. It helps heal the gut mucosa, improve the absorption of nutrients, and stimulate the lymphatic system. The tea helps move fluid through and out of the body, so you may urinate more, which is a good sign. Here's how to prepare this pleasant-tasting savory tea:

Prime Tea

Boil 4 to 5 cups of water in a pot.

As the water is heating, add the following to the pot:

½ teaspoon cumin seeds
½ teaspoon coriander seeds
½ teaspoon fennel seeds

Additional options:

- ½ teaspoon manjistha powder, if you have lymphatic backup as indicated by the Fake Fat quiz on page 88. (You can add this to the steeped, strained tea afterward, since it is a powder and doesn't require straining.)

- ½ teaspoon fenugreek seeds, if you are having a lot of excess gas production.

- ½ to 1 inch peeled fresh ginger, for people who want to increase their agni even further (some people have a particularly hard time igniting that digestive fire). Just add it while the water is boiling. For a stronger ginger flavor, you can keep the fresh ginger in the thermos; for a weaker ginger flavor, strain it out with the other ingredients.

Let the water boil for five to ten minutes with the seeds, depending on how strong you want your tea to be. Afterward, strain the seeds out of the tea, then pour the tea into an insulated vessel (like a thermos) to keep it hot all day. If you have a tea ball, use it for less cleanup. Then sip the tea throughout the day until it's all gone. Try to finish it before 6 p.m., so you don't have to use the bathroom multiple times during the night.

This tea is powerful for several reasons. One of the most straightforward is temperature. Think about how you clean things. Hot water always works better than cold. Just as during a facial you may steam your face to clean out your pores because heat opens pores, in the same way, heat opens up the channels inside the body for more efficient waste removal.

The body is like a vast network of roads. Some of these roads are like multilane interstate highways. Some are like two-lane highways, some are county roads connecting small towns, and still others are like little dirt paths. The roads consist of your major arteries and veins, the channels of lymph that flow just under your skin, even the little microscopic channels in the gaps between cells. These channels also include the *nadis* and *srotas* that Ayurvedic medicine recognizes. All of these channels are responsible for moving fluid like blood and lymph, distributing nutrients to organs, and eliminating waste from the body. They travel to and from your heart, lungs, liver, and glands and to the farthest reaches of your body, from brain to pinky toe.

But often these channels get clogged, like a freeway pile-up, a mudslide across a highway, or a fallen tree over a residential street. The simple warmth from the tea is a vasodilator, opening blood vessels and lymph vessels to widen those freeway lanes and clear the way. It's like building an extra lane to accommodate construction, or widening a narrow road.

It isn't just the warmth that benefits. Otherwise, you could drink any tea, or even hot water, for that matter. Another reason the tea is so powerful is the particular spices it contains. Cumin, coriander, and fennel are three of the most powerful spices for stimulating the digestion, increasing the metabolism, and waking up a dull and sluggish gut to get things moving again.

- *Cumin* is an ancient remedy for indigestion, gas, and other digestive issues. It includes potent antioxidants and iron, as well as fiber, and it stimulates the enzymes in the body that facilitate strong digestion. Studies have shown that cumin also soothes inflamed mucous membranes in the digestive tract and improves bowel function.[1]

- *Coriander* is a digestive aid with a pleasant nutty taste, and its properties are enhanced by heat. In Ayurveda, coriander is used to treat many intestinal disorders because it relieves gas, indigestion, and spasms, and it reduces inflammation. It has also been shown to inhibit the joint swelling associated with rheumatoid arthritis.[2]

- *Fennel* is a remedy for colic, irritable bowel syndrome, and other painful digestive issues because it relaxes the smooth muscle in the digestive tract. It's also good for relieving excess gas and indigestion and encouraging the body to burn fat. It contains phytoestrogens, so it's great for women having hormonal issues, and it also tends to suppress excessive appetite in a balanced way. Fennel is particularly good at moving lymph out of the body to reduce Fake Fat. When you chew a few seeds, it has the added benefit of being a breath freshener.

It is truly an eye-opening experience to make this tea part of your daily life. As you work through the first stage of this plan, you will notice a sense of warmth growing in your belly, your agni. This is the energy that absorbs nutrients, assimilates them into the body, and burns off toxins and excess fat. If your digestion is weak, you feel cold all the time, and you feel lethargic, this tea will help because it increases the energy of agni and at the same time begins to reduce inflammation in the body.

By the way, this recipe often gets passed on to my patients' friends and family members because it is so good at soothing the digestive system. I've even had people give it as a gift during the holidays. Why keep the goodness all to yourself?

Triphala

This is one of my favorite parts of The Prime. Triphala really is the closest thing I know to a miracle cure. It's widely available; it is made from three berries that are dried and ground up, so it is a whole food product; and the changes it causes in the body are dramatic. You may remember that my family used to eat some of these berries, often pickled, as a condiment with our meals. You can't find them easily that way in the United States, but fortunately they are available in dried, powdered form, so you can still enjoy all of triphala's benefits. Though the name may be new to you, or sound Seuss-like, triphala is not some weird, dangerous herbal remedy. It's just berries. And the amount in a capsule's worth of powder is equal to less than one berry, at most. In my clinic, we often give spoonfuls of triphala powder, and we don't worry about "overdosing" because that would be like overdosing on, for instance, blueberries. Pretty hard to do.

Triphala is a fantastic combination of foods. It has a mild laxative effect, but it is such a good colon cleanser because it heals the mucosal lining and the nerves in the gut, so you can experience normal peristalsis again. Instead of forcing your colon to expel its contents, triphala helps the colon do what it is naturally supposed to do. Your gut remembers how it is supposed to work because the triphala is repairing the injury. Unlike a laxative that you have to take forever, you can take triphala for a while, then stop for a bit because it has already done its work. That being said, I've taken triphala for fifteen years. I don't take it for its laxative effects. I take it because life is stressful every single day, and those stresses send a lot of signals that interfere with your ENS. For example, I have to travel a lot. When I can't get the best food, the antioxidants in triphala help me manage some of the chronic wear and tear in my gut associated with travel.

As it is available today, triphala is labeled in terms of milligrams. Aim for 1,000 milligrams per day to start. Depending on which brand you buy, this may involve taking one or two tablets in the evening, about an hour before bedtime. (I use and recommend Organic Digest Tone Triphala Plus by VPK—see the Resources section for more information). If, within a week, you are not having one good bowel movement every day, increase your dosage to 2,000 milligrams per day. If, after another week, things still aren't "moving along," increase the dosage to 3,000 milligrams. You can go as high as 4,000 milligrams quite safely—remember, triphala is just dried berries.

The longer it takes for triphala to work, the more you need it and the longer you should stay in Stage One of The Prime. The amount of time it takes to start working for you depends on your gut IQ, so if your score on the Gut IQ Test showed that your gut needs a longer education, be prepared to allow triphala some time to work its powerful effects on you. You need your colon working efficiently for the remainder of The Prime to be effective.

Once your digestion is moving, you will begin to notice a metabolic shift in your body. You will begin to detoxify more efficiently. Triphala works so well for detoxification because of the triple action of the three berries it contains: amlaki (amla), haritaki, and bibhitaki. Let's look more closely at them.

> ### ANCIENT WISDOM
>
> Triphala is so widely revered in India that there is an old saying that goes, "Even if you don't have a mother, if you have triphala, you have nothing to worry about." An exaggeration, perhaps, but indicative of how powerful and health-enhancing triphala can be.

Amlaki (or Amla)

Amlaki, also called Indian gooseberry or amla, is one of the most potent antioxidants out there and one of the most important medicinal plants used in Ayurvedic medicine. The fruit is an excellent anti-inflammatory and anti-fever agent, has a mild laxative effect, and is even being studied for its anti-cancer properties.[3] It's really good at helping to reduce inflammation and stabilizing blood sugar. Some studies say it is as effective as oral medications for the treatment of diabetes.[4] I think that's pretty impressive.

There are two key reasons amlaki is so good at fighting diabetes. First, it helps normalize blood sugar and stabilizes appetite and mood, so you're not fighting the peaks and valleys that can trigger binge eating. Second, it encourages the body to build lean muscle mass, which helps regulate blood sugar more efficiently. Amla fundamentally begins to alter your body, even without a change to your diet or exercise routine. I also like amla because it helps the liver work more efficiently and also provides antioxidants to nourish the body during detoxification. Amla helps balance some of the acidic properties of food as well. It has an alkaline effect on the tissues of the body after being metabolized, helping to reduce the impact of inflammation. It's one of the best things you can add to your daily routine, and having it in your daily triphala supplement really can change your body over time in profound ways.

Haritaki

Haritaki is a berry that is particularly good at removing toxins from the colon. This helps nurture a healthier balance of bacteria in your colon, discouraging the microorganisms that feed on sugar and encouraging those that are more beneficial for overall health. Fewer toxins means a stronger immune system and stronger digestion. Even more striking, research shows that haritaki has a significant hypolipidemic effect. That means it gets rid of fat, helps lower cholesterol and triglycerides, and helps boost the good cholesterol that protects you from heart disease.[5] A study of haritaki also demonstrated its antibacterial and antifungal properties against such undesirable pathogens as *E. coli*, fungal infections of the skin, and internal bacterial overgrowth resulting in issues such as chronic ulcers.[6]

Bibhitaki

Finally, bibhitaki (also called *Terminalia belerica*) is a berry that breaks down fat and opens up your lymphatic channels. Fake Fat begins to dissipate as your lymph moves toxins out and flushes excess fluid accumulation. Bibhitaki can also move congestion and has traditionally been used against asthma and as an expectorant to clear the lungs. Like haritaki, it also has a hypolipidemic effect, lowering cholesterol and fat in the liver and heart, and it also has a blood-pressure-lowering effect. Some research even suggests that bibhitaki could fight HIV and malaria. I think of bibhitaki as a sort of vacuum cleaner suction for toxins. In Sanskrit, there is a saying about bibhitaki, that when you take it, disease cannot come near you.

That sums up the wonder that is triphala. If I were ever stuck on a desert island and I could take only one single supplement with me, triphala would be it. Triphala aids so many different things in the body that it really is one of my favorite herbal remedies.

Fiber Therapy

The last thing you are going to do in Stage One is take some fiber. That's pretty normal, right? A lot of people take fiber for constipation, but most Americans are grossly deficient in fiber, which is likely one of the major reasons that sluggish digestion and constipation are such common problems. Women need at least 25 grams of fiber every day, and men need 38 grams, but most adults get only 15 grams at most.

There is an easy way to remedy this issue, and it doesn't involve heaping bowls of twiggy cereal. Every other evening, with your triphala, put 1 teaspoon each of psyllium husks and ground flax seeds in a 12-ounce glass of warm or room-temperature water. Stir it briskly with a spoon and drink it down quickly because it can get thick if you leave it in the water too long. If you need to follow it with more water, go ahead. That's all you have to do. In thirty seconds, you will have dramatically boosted your daily fiber intake.

The reason I have you taking fiber every other day rather than every day is that the fiber can slightly interfere with the absorption of the triphala, so every other day, I want you to take triphala alone. You will still get the benefits of both with an every-other-day regimen.

Don't worry about the taste. It's nutty and a bit grainy, nothing offensive there. And the effect this will have on your digestive system is pretty amazing. The bulk you are adding to your digestive system suctions out the waste for speedy and easy elimination. This fiber is also food for your internal microbiome—the good gut bacteria that will encourage better dietary choices and fat loss. Fiber encourages the proliferation of good bacteria and helps whisk away the bad bacteria that are dying off as you get healthier and your body sheds and discards them.

IF YOU NEED A FIBER ADJUSTMENT

Most people who are fiber-deficient need to step up to a healthful amount gradually because at first, your gut flora is oriented toward sugar and fat rather than fiber and it won't know what to do with large amounts of fiber. This can cause unpleasant (although temporary) side effects, such as bloating and gas, but as fiber is a prebiotic (food for the good bacteria in your digestive tract), this will soon change. Remember that any initial uncomfortable feelings are a sign that your gut bacteria are changing. If you notice any of these symptoms, just lower your dose a bit—start with 1/2 teaspoon each of psyllium husks and ground flax seeds. Soon you'll tolerate fiber easily. It will make you feel great because your digestion will no longer be sluggish and uncomfortable.

Priming Your Body in Stage One: How You Will Feel

You are going to start feeling better as your body releases the toxins it may have been storing for a long time. As you learned in the last chapter, you will also likely feel some minor detox symptoms (see the Stage One Detox Box on page 140) that are somewhat uncomfortable, but these are clear signs that the process is working. As toxins clear out of your body, you will notice increased mental clarity. Your sleep will become deeper and more restorative. You may feel lighter and more energetic, or you may begin to feel tired or sluggish, or notice some breakouts on your face or even the occasional headache or joint pain.

Don't be deterred by some uncomfortable feelings, both physical and emotional. These are a natural part of detoxification. Remember that as your body gets rid of the toxins or *ama*, the bad bacteria are dying off and your entire system is shifting. As the detox symptoms resolve, you will probably notice that your cravings begin to evolve. You may want less sugar or fat. Processed food may begin to taste strange or unpleasant. In fact, one of the biggest changes my clients report is the development of taste aversions to things they once craved. This is an important development and the first sign that your ENS is communicating with you again, telling you that it is ready for some changes. Some of my patients tell me that they will eat, for example, a candy bar in the afternoon because they are in the habit of doing so, and suddenly it will make them sick. That fast-food burger may trigger a migraine, even though you never realized before that it was a migraine trigger.

Detoxification reduces the cause-and-effect time lag between a food and a reaction. How your body responds to the foods you eat will become more obvious to you. You may then be in a better and stronger position to decide to avoid certain things, when you realize that the pain and discomfort they cause aren't worth the momentary enjoyment of eating them. Many of my patients report, even in the first thirty days, that they decide to avoid things that they suddenly realize are problematic for them.

This happens because, as the body gets rid of the junk clogging the system, it becomes more sensitive to what you put into it. I won't tell you to stop eating candy bars or cheeseburgers, but if your body tells you to stop, then listen to it and act according to what feels right and good for you. This is the beginning of a level of body awareness you may never have experienced before.

Stick with it because it's only going to get better and better.

How Long to Continue

You already have an idea from the Gut IQ Test what track (Fast, Moderate, Gentle) you want to take and how much time you should spend in Stage One. However, this is only a guideline. You should stay here until your body has reaped all the available benefits from Stage One. When you reach a new equilibrium and your detox symptoms abate, you are ready to move to the next stage.

STAGE ONE DETOX BOX

Your detox in Stage One is mild, but you still may notice some uncomfortable symptoms, such as skin breakouts, weird-smelling sweat or urine, fatigue, headaches, joint pain, brain fog, or irritability. If these are uncomfortable, here are some management strategies:

- **GO SLOWER.** Add only one step at a time for two weeks, and then add the next step. Even though these are pretty gentle ingredients, if you have never done a detox before or you have accumulated a large toxin load, your organs need some time to wake up and adjust.

- **DRINK PLENTY OF WATER.** In addition to Prime Tea, make sure you are drinking another liter (about 4 cups) of warm or lukewarm water throughout the day. Your body needs help flushing out the toxins.

- **INCREASE YOUR FIBER INTAKE.** If your body has adjusted to the full dose of psyllium husks and flax seeds, then go ahead and increase it to 2 teaspoons each and eventually, even 3 teaspoons. Fiber absorbs toxins and sweeps them away so they aren't reabsorbed in your gut and pulled back into your bloodstream for your liver to process again. Fiber helps you catch the ama and eliminate it more efficiently. Just as in every other step, go slowly and pay attention to how your body tolerates each change.

- **REST MORE.** Even though you can't see the energy being used by your body, trust me, your body is working hard. Just as you need more rest when you are doing more mental or physical work, you need more rest when you are doing more biochemical work. Even going to bed one hour earlier can make a big difference.

CRUSH CRAVINGS (NO WILLPOWER REQUIRED)

We are going to up the ante in Stage Two by targeting your cravings for foods that are not helping your health. These are the addictive foods we talked about earlier that trigger your neuroadaptation mechanisms so that you become dependent on them. These are the foods that cause your body to downregulate your dopamine receptors, to deal with those unnatural pleasure spikes. In Stage Two, we are going to help your body calm down and reorient, so you can get pleasure from foods that are also nutrient-rich and natural (rather than highly processed and full of chemicals). Here is how we'll do it:

STAGE TWO SNAPSHOT

- **CURB CRAVINGS WITH ASHWAGANDHA.** Take 400 to 500 milligrams every morning with breakfast and every evening before dinner (try to take it before 6 p.m.).

- **BALANCE YOUR BRAIN WITH BRAHMI.** Take 400 to 500 milligrams every morning with breakfast and every evening before dinner (try to take it before 6 p.m.). Please take Brahmi and ashwagandha together, as they act synergistically.

- **START THE DAY WITH PRIME JUICE.** Fresh vegetable juice floods your body with antioxidants, vitamins, and other phytonutrients without the added burden of raw vegetable fiber (which the juicer takes out), which can be difficult to digest when your gut needs healing. Prime Juice can also be an excellent response to sugar cravings because of the concentration of nutrients, since sugar cravings are often really just cravings for nutrients. Have this before you eat breakfast three to five mornings per week. (You may find you won't need as much breakfast, so pay attention to how you feel after drinking the juice.) This juice is most potent within twenty minutes of preparation, but if you know you tend to have a midafternoon sugar craving, save some to have later. It will still be highly effective around 2 or 3 p.m. when most people get their sugar cravings.

- **SEAL THE DEAL WITH PRIME BROTH.** Prime Broth helps heal a damaged or leaky gut lining, and it fills you up with nourishing minerals and vitamins. This is essential for building up your nutrient reserves as you detoxify, so your body works better and you have more energy. Prime Broth can complement your lunch, but it is not a meal replacement for lunch. Your agni is highest in the middle of the day, and this is the best time to eat your largest meal. In the evening, your agni is lower and you may find that after a bowl of Prime Broth, you're not hungry for much more. I recommend Prime Broth for or with dinner three to five nights per week. If you really love it, go ahead and have some with lunch, too.

- **WRITE IT DOWN.** Journal your cravings. You will start a cravings journal during this stage, to help yourself become more self-aware.

Continue Stage One's Healthy Habits:

- **DRY-BRUSH** your skin before your morning shower.
- **MAKE YOUR TEA** and sip on it throughout the day.
- **TAKE TRIPHALA:** 1,000 milligrams of triphala every night, or more if you have already increased your dosage in Stage One.
- **TAKE FIBER** every other day: Mix 1 teaspoon each of ground flax seeds and psyllium husks (or the amount you worked up to in Stage One) into a glass of room-temperature water and drink.

Now let's look more closely at each element that makes this stage so powerful.

One of the best ways I know to normalize unwanted neuroadaptation in the brain is through the use of an herb called ashwagandha. Also called Indian ginseng (despite its name, it is related not to ginseng but instead to the tomato plant), ashwagandha is a popular medicinal herb in India and an excellent remedy for stress, low energy, and cravings, especially for sugar.[1] Research supports many health benefits and no risks from ashwagandha.[2] It is one of only a few known herbal *adaptogens*,[3] meaning it specifically helps the body adapt to stress in a healthy rather than dysfunctional way.[4] It also strengthens an exhausted nervous system and calms emotions. This is the herb to counteract anxiety, agitation, stress, and PMS. Now that your gut is able to absorb ashwagandha, it can have a truly potent effect on you.

And now that you are winning the battle of the gut, you can launch the battle for the brain.

As your body detoxifies, you are moving into a new homeostasis, with less inflammation and fewer toxins. Your brain is changing, too—you experience fewer extreme dopamine spikes, and your brain notices this shift. While some people experience decreased cravings while detoxifying, at first there is often a period when these cravings increase. This is because, as you continue with The Prime, the impact you are making on your body becomes more and more profound, and sometimes the brain fights back, trying to reclaim the older patterns it had established because of neuroadaptation. This is why ashwagandha is so crucial at this stage. It furthers the normalization of general brain function.

This can also cause you a little bit of personal confusion—I don't forbid any foods, and you may find that you crave the junk food you have been eating but also don't want to eat it. It's a strange feeling, but it is a sign that your body is slowly readjusting. If you do eat junk food, pay attention to how you feel afterward. You may soon realize that the way it makes you feel isn't worth the momentary pleasure. You may find that you don't really want to eat it after all, or that you want only a smaller amount. Remember earlier when I explained how your gut bacteria can control your cravings? They send signals to your brain that tell you to eat the foods they want—the foods that got you into a toxic inflammatory state. Ashwagandha works with the brain to reroute those messages to the junk mail pile. Those cravings, which are signs of withdrawal from addictive foods and the dying off of the bad gut bacteria that need sugar to survive, won't feel as powerful or compelling within your system when you have ashwagandha on board to help.

Brahmi

Brahmi (also called *Bacopa monniera*) is another herb common in India. It is a ground cover–like creeping plant and has been a medicinal herb there since ancient times. It is named after Brahman, the Hindu deity that represents universal creativity and consciousness, and Brahmi is, not coincidentally, powerful at improving every aspect of the brain. It is often served as a cooked vegetable, alone or in soup, used raw in salads, or made into pickles. In the United States, it is primarily available as the dried ground whole plant, in capsule form, but it is still the same plant. It's best to take it with ashwagandha since they act synergistically. The ideal time to take both is in the morning and again before dinner (and before 6 p.m.), when your body tends to have an energy slump and you're particularly susceptible to cravings.

As a neurologist, I like Brahmi for its effects on the brain. In Ayurveda, it is considered a "brain tonic" because it has an overall balancing effect on cognitive function, but specifically, it helps normalize the release of dopamine and correct the pleasure circuits that have been overloaded and exhausted. In Ayurveda, we use Brahmi to help with addictions, Parkinson's disease, epilepsy, and a host of other neurological conditions. Its effect is both gentle and noticeable. This herb is also so powerful that many of my patients tell me that about halfway through The Prime, they are finally able to quit smoking, or they decide to give up alcohol or recreational drugs. This is a happy side effect of the rebalancing of the brain's neurochemistry that Brahmi supports.

Brahmi is also traditionally used to improve memory,[5] concentration, and even IQ. It's the smart herb that can help you be smarter about what you choose to eat because Brahmi helps the brain coordinate all its functions. It brings orderliness to all the brain's pathways, so it positively influences the symptoms of Alzheimer's disease, ADHD, autism, and even drug addiction. It also helps suppress the appetite. I think it is amazing how nature provides us with the remedy for addiction, but Brahmi isn't just for brain dysfunction. It is for brain maximization.

Prime Juice

While ashwagandha and Brahmi work on your brain, Prime Juice and Prime Broth work on your body. Cravings can sometimes be signals of malnourishment. In the Western world, we typically don't have a problem getting enough calories. Yet we have a big problem getting enough nutrients. We are not undernourished; we are malnourished. It can be hard to know when a craving comes from real need or when it comes from an addictive response, but both Prime Juice and Prime Broth are interventions I have found to be highly effective for stemming cravings due to malnourishment.

Prime Juice is an excellent remedy for malnourishment because it contains concentrated vitamins, antioxidants, and other valuable components of vegetables and fruits in an easy-to-digest form. The best way to prepare it is with a juicer. If you don't have one, this can be a great investment in your health. Although some people make juice in the blender by liquefying the ingredients with water, I prefer a juicer because when agni is low, it is hard to process large amounts of raw food. Removing the fiber at this stage will make the nutrients from the vegetables much easier to absorb and less stressful on the digestion. (Don't get confused about the fiber you take at night versus fiber from the vegetables you juice—raw vegetables are difficult to digest and that can make their nutrients difficult to absorb. The juice makes this easier—you get the more easily absorbed nutrients without the potentially troublesome raw vegetable fiber. The pure supplemental fiber you take at night serves the important purpose of binding toxins and sweeping them from the body.)

WARNING FOR THOSE WITH HYPERTHYROIDISM

If you have been diagnosed with hyperthyroidism, also known as Graves' disease, you should be cautious about using ashwagandha and Brahmi. The doses I recommend are pretty small, but these two herbs are known to potentially increase thyroid function so that the thyroid operates more normally. This is great for people with a sluggish thyroid (which is more common), but for those with hyperthyroidism who typically overproduce thyroid hormone, these herbs may be contraindicated. The challenging part of making Ayurvedic recommendations for an isolated diagnosis such as hyperthyroidism is that there are times that we use herbs such as Brahmi and ashwagandha in the treatment for it and other times when we would not—it is individualized to the needs of the person. This may sound counterintuitive, but because these herbs have dynamic roles in the body, coordinating the function of multiple organs, for some they help control certain aspects of hyperthyroidism, but for others they may aggravate them. If you have hyperthyroidism, I would recommend working with an Ayurvedic practitioner to see if it is appropriate to take this low dose of ashwagandha and Brahmi. Otherwise, check with your regular doctor, who can monitor your thyroid function while you are on the program.

Prime Juice works best in the morning before breakfast or in the afternoon if sugar cravings surface. Prepare a juice that is made from 90 percent vegetables and 10 percent fruit. The small amount of fruit makes the juice taste nice but doesn't contribute to a blood sugar spike, which can sometimes happen when you juice a fruit but don't eat the fiber.

I recommend two different recipes, depending on the season and how you are feeling. For each, run all the ingredients through a juicer and drink immediately, or drink half and save the other half in an airtight container in the refrigerator for a midafternoon energy slump.

Prime Juice #1

Use this juice when you are feeling anxious and ungrounded, or sluggish and unmotivated. This juice is also good for fall, winter, and spring, or whenever the weather is cooler.

Makes 1 serving

1 cucumber
1 apple, seeds removed
1 handful fresh spinach
¼ head purple cabbage
1 carrot
1 beet
1 lemon (you can use the entire thing, but cut it into quarters before juicing)
1 inch peeled fresh ginger
Optional: ½ to 1 teaspoon spirulina powder, stirred into the juice after preparing. The taste is strong so if you want to try it, start on the low side and work up to a full teaspoon.

Chop the vegetables to fit your juicer. Put all ingredients through a juicer and drink immediately. (Do not use a blender.)

Prime Juice #2

Use this juice when you are feeling irritable, acidic, or overheated. This juice is also good for summer, or whenever the weather is hot.

Makes 1 serving

1 cucumber
1 celery stalk
1 apple, seeds removed
½ head purple cabbage
2 to 3 kale leaves
1 handful cilantro
½ lemon, including the peel
Optional: ½ to 1 teaspoon spirulina powder, stirred into the juice after preparing. Again, the taste is strong, so if you want to try it, start on the low side and work up to a full teaspoon.

Chop the vegetables to fit your juicer. Put all ingredients through a juicer and drink immediately. (Do not use a blender.)

Both versions of this juice contain pure and absorbable nutrition, and they can also help minimize detoxification symptoms.

Prime Broth

Bone broth is an old remedy for the common cold, but it is also a highly mineralizing, nourishing, and anti-inflammatory food.[6] It is basically just broth made by boiling bones and other parts of the animal that are also rich in nutrients, with or without meat on them. In general, especially for weight loss, Ayurvedic medicine does not recommend eating meat except in the form of a broth, since bone broth is digestible and nutrient-rich. Bone broth contains dissolved minerals that can replenish a malnourished body. The amino acids in it help rebuild muscle and connective tissue. Glycine, in particular, helps heal the gut lining when it is damaged and leaky, and there is even some evidence that glycine calms the brain and increases alertness. It is also a detoxifier, specifically in the liver.[7] The amino acid proline, also in bone broth, may help clear the arteries of deposits and clean the blood. Finally, the marrow from the bones is easy to absorb and is a dense source of nutrition.

A lot of people who are overweight are also malnourished. We have to fix that, or the body won't have the nutrients necessary to heal properly in Stage Three of The Prime. Prime Broth is one of the best ways to reverse malnourishment.

A SPECIAL NOTE TO VEGETARIANS

I get a lot of pushback about Prime Broth from my vegetarian and vegan patients. The concept can be tough for them, and I totally understand this. It was certainly tough for me at first, too. I had been a vegetarian and I didn't like the idea of eating animal products. Because of my digestive issues, however, my own Ayurvedic physician recommended that I start bone broth to help me heal my gut. I protested for almost two years until I realized I really did need the extra support. Finally, I relented at the constant insistence of my Ayurvedic physician, and the effects were profound.

Today, I would say I am 90 percent vegan. The only exceptions are lassi and ghee (you'll learn more about those later in this book), and Prime Broth when I am feeling depleted. I especially use Prime Broth as medicine when I travel because it takes a lot out of me. I only make broth from humanely treated animals, raised organically, and before I drink it, I say a little prayer of gratitude, acknowledging the exchange of energy. I have tremendous gratitude and bless the sacrifice made on my behalf.

In Western culture, we don't tend to look at meat as medicine. We see it as an everyday food. This leads to our culture eating way too much of it on a regular basis, and not for the right purposes. In Ayurvedic medicine, bone marrow is one of the last tissues to be formed, so it's extremely nutrient-rich in an accessible way. Muscle meat is hard to break down and it requires a strong digestion. If you don't have strong digestion, your body will have a difficult time extracting nutrients from muscle meat. On the other hand, Prime Broth is easy to absorb. It also promotes the type of gut flora that increases health.

Although I still don't like the idea of eating animals, Prime Broth is so healing and mineralizing that I believe it is worth making an exception. If you are willing to try it, it can make a big difference in the speed of your digestive healing. Once you are finished with The Prime and you are nourished, you don't have to continue the Prime Broth. If you like the effects, I suggest you continue to use it in place of meat in your diet.

If you are morally opposed to bone broth, however, I certainly won't tell you to go against your feelings. It took me two years to agree to it, and I don't believe that anyone should take any action they believe to be wrong. If this is you, just go with the Prime Juice and the other elements of this stage.

I prefer to use poultry bones because bones from larger animals tend to have more concentrated toxins and larger animals tend to be more frequently mistreated. As long as you find bones from a healthy animal, preferably organic and grass fed or free range, your Prime Broth will be therapeutic. Also use organic vegetables, if you can.

I suggest you make this broth in a slow cooker because cooking it slowly at a low temperature is important for extracting the bone marrow. However, you could do this in a stockpot on the stove. You would need to keep it there for eight to ten hours at a low temperature, however, and most people don't have time to keep an eye on the stove for that long. I find a slow cooker to be much more convenient.

Here is my recipe:

Prime Broth

1 chicken or small turkey carcass, or 3 to 6 pounds (depending on
   how big your slow cooker is) of any meaty bones, with marrow
2 onions, quartered
4 celery stalks, cut into large chunks (you may include the leaves)
2 large carrots, cut into chunks
¼ cup (for 3 pounds of bones) to ½ cup (for 6 pounds of bones)
   apple cider vinegar (I prefer raw versions, such as Bragg's)
Enough water to fill the slow cooker up to about 2 inches from
   the top
1 tablespoon Himalayan or other pure salt
Optional: A few chicken feet, for extra gelatin in the broth
   (these are often available from the meat counter at the
   grocery store—try it if you aren't squeamish)

Put the bones and vegetables in a slow cooker. Drizzle the vinegar over the bones; then add the water and sea salt. Cook on low for 24 to 48 hours. Strain out the bones and vegetables and store the broth in the refrigerator for up to a week, or in individual portions in the freezer for up to six months. Note: when the Prime Broth is chilled, it will turn into a thick gelatin, but it will liquefy again when you heat it up. Also, you can remove the fat that coagulates on top of the Prime Broth when chilled, if you like a leaner broth; leave it in if you like a richer broth. You can also freeze Prime Broth for future use. Make a big batch every few weeks and you will always have it handy for when you need it.

You can sip Prime Broth on its own, but the way I prefer to use it is as a base for soup. I'll eat the soup as a starter course to my main meal of the day, lunch, or alone as a light dinner:

Prime Broth Variation: Vegetable Soup

Sometimes, you may want something a little more interesting than Prime Broth. In that case, you can also add veggies to make this a hearty and filling meal. Here is my recipe. You can use any green veggies you have on hand, or that are fresh and seasonal.

Serves 2, but you can double or triple this recipe if you want to make it ahead for the week

1 cup Prime Broth

1 cup water

1 cup chopped green vegetables (use what you have or what is seasonal, such as chopped kale, spinach, zucchini, green beans, broccoli, asparagus)

1 teaspoon or more of any spices you like (In the next stage, you will be making Prime Curry Powder, and it is very good in this soup. If you want to jump ahead to page 166 and make that recipe earlier, I won't object. Add about ½ teaspoon per serving, or more to taste.)

Combine everything in a saucepan and bring to a boil. Cook for 10 to 12 minutes once it's boiling. Eat as is, or blend for a puréed soup.

PURCHASING BONE BROTH

If you don't have the time or inclination to make your own bone broth, you can buy this type of traditional bone broth from companies that use healthy animals. This is not the same as boxed or canned broth from the grocery store. Those are not real bone broth. They may contain a small amount, but they are nothing like what you can make at home, or what you can buy from select sources. I was lucky enough to find a place that makes it near where I live— The Brothery in Carlsbad, California. Now I no longer make my own broth. They deliver nationwide, but see if you can find a similar local place. Your local farmer's market or food co-op may have a source.

Cravings Journal

The final step for this part of the program is to start a cravings journal. I won't make you write down everything you eat, but what I would like you to write down (in a notebook, or even in a note-taking app on your phone) is your cravings. Keep track of what time you have them, what you crave, and how you are feeling at that moment. This can be an excellent way to notice patterns in your cravings so you can be aware that they are not random. This can also help you take steps to thwart them (such as a glass of Prime Juice or a cup of Prime Broth thirty minutes before you typically have cravings).

Finally, doing this can help you recognize when your cravings are really emotional ones, so you can begin to feed yourself with things other than food. If you always get cravings when you are bored or lonely or angry, then your body is trying to resolve your issues, but you may be misinterpreting the message. This is the format I like to use:

Date	Time	What I'm Craving	How I'm Feeling	What Do I Really Want?

Priming Your Body in Stage Two: How You Will Feel

Many of the detoxification symptoms you may have been feeling during Stage One are likely fading away. That's because you are doing so much to improve your nutritional status, which makes your detoxification pathways more efficient at clearing the toxins out. You are feeling better and everything seems to be working better. This is great. If you aren't yet feeling this, stay at this stage until you do.

CRAVING CALMER: CARDAMOM PODS

One of the nice things about Stage Two is that you won't have as many uncomfortable symptoms as you did in Stage One (or will in Stage Three). You are nourishing your body so fully now that your detox symptoms have likely abated. There is one exception, however—sugar cravings. For some, sugar cravings are exceptionally powerful and resistant. Those sugar-loving gut bacteria don't want to die! This stage is particularly geared toward reducing sugar cravings, but sometimes you will get breakthrough cravings that you want to control but can't. These sugar cravings can really derail your good intentions, especially during certain times of the month if you're female. When your weight is normal and you are healthy, it won't hurt you to have a sweet snack (made from real food) when you have a craving. But if you are at the point where you know that sugar will just set you off, try a trick that works well for me: cardamom pods.

Cardamom pods are a useful weapon against sugar cravings, which is why I suggest keeping them handy during Stage Two. Unlike the cardamom seeds you use in your tea, these include the pods they grow in. If sugar cravings feel unmanageable but you don't want to eat something sweet because you know you won't feel good afterward, just pop a cardamom pod in your mouth. Suck on it until your craving passes, and then spit it out. Cardamom ties into your dopamine reward system, satiating your sugar craving without providing you with sugar that will overload your dopamine receptors. Look for organic versions at health food stores such as Whole Foods and Sprouts, or order them online.

Cardamom pods can serve you even after you are done with The Prime. I like these, especially, during my menstrual cycle, a natural time of detoxification, but also a time that can feel stressful and trigger cravings for comfort food. I get strong sugar cravings then, as well as when I am traveling, so I always keep cardamom pods with me.

Sugar cravings are also quite common for many between 2 and 6 p.m. Ayurveda has an explanation for this: this is the time of day when your body is at its weakest and you are most prone to addictive triggers. If you know you are prone to afternoon sugar cravings, in addition to the other Prime suggestions of this stage, you can use cardamom pods for prevention. Just pop a pod in your mouth at 2 p.m. and suck on it for about an hour. This should get you past the worst part. If you still feel the craving, pop another one into your mouth. At first use, you may still want something sweet. If you've tried cardamom and you still want it, go ahead and have it, but notice whether you are inclined to eat less of that sweet snack than you may have before. Next time, you may not want it at all.

How Long to Continue

It is extremely important to improve your nutritional status before moving on to Stage Three. If you need to spend a little more time at Stage Two, that is totally fine. In Stage Three, you are going to supercharge your detox pathways in your liver, and your body has to have the stored nutrients to support this process so the toxins can get all the way out. These are signs that you are ready to move on:

- Your energy is improving—you may even notice that your body wants to move more.
- You have more mental clarity.
- You have noticed a spontaneous reduction in cravings.
- Your mood feels more even-keeled and you're not having as many highs and lows throughout the day.

IGNITE ENERGY AND FAT

We've swept up and taken out the trash. We've nourished the body and thwarted some of those nasty cravings. Now it's time to go deeper. In Stage Three of The Prime, we are going to start squeezing out the junk that has accumulated at a deeper level. After you take out the trash, you can get down on your hands and knees and scrub out the grime (metaphorically speaking). The second thing we are going to do at this point is ignite the digestive fire. I've already explained what agni is, but as a reminder, agni in the digestive system burns food for energy and agni in the liver incinerates toxicity. You want both fires to be burning strong and hot so you can get the most nutrients out of your food to support detoxification, and to get those toxins out with the utmost efficiency. It is important to do these two steps simultaneously because a strong digestive fire will help burn off the sludge that guggul, in particular, will pull out of your system and drop into your digestive tract.

STAGE THREE SNAPSHOT

- **GUGGUL IT.** Take 500 milligrams every morning and evening. (Later in this chapter, I will explain if and when you should increase or decrease this dose.)

- **SPICE UP YOUR LIFE WITH PRIME CURRY POWDER.** Make up a fresh batch every month and use it in the foods you cook or stir it into room-temperature or warm water. Aim for 1/2 to 1 teaspoon per day, added to your diet in whatever way you choose, as a minimum. You can use more—up to 3 teaspoons per day total, preferably divided between lunch and dinner. (You could use it for breakfast, too, if you like a savory breakfast.)

- **FLUSH YOUR GUT WITH GINGER.** The Ginger Gut Flush is a powerful digestion stimulator. Just chew on a piece of this specially prepared fresh ginger with lunch and dinner. If you have a lot of gas, constipation, and bloating, increase to two to three pieces with lunch and dinner. If you tend to have heartburn or get rashes or become irritable easily, you may want to just try ginger in a supplement form. In this case, take 500 milligrams with lunch and dinner. If this causes you to feel too hot (i.e., you notice more heartburn or more rashes or feel more irritable), then skip the ginger. It's not for you.

Continue These Stage One and Two Habits

Don't be deterred as these steps add up. Each of these things takes just minutes, some even just seconds, and they can be done all together (like taking supplements) or as part of meals or things you do while doing something else (like sipping tea). It may look like a long list, but as these habits become integrated into your life, they won't seem to take any time at all.

- **DRY-BRUSH YOUR SKIN** before your morning shower. Dry-brushing is even more important now as the detox accelerates, so keep it up!

- **DRINK YOUR TEA.** Keep making and sipping on it throughout the day.

- **TAKE TRIPHALA** at the level you were taking before, unless you are currently taking less than 1,000 milligrams. In this case, it is a good time to increase your dosage to 1,000 milligrams per night because your colon is putting in a lot of work in Stage Three and can use the boost.

- **TAKE FIBER** every other day. Continue with your Stage Two dosage, unless you are taking less than 1 teaspoon each of ground flax seeds and psyllium husks. If so, this is a good time to move up to 1 teaspoon each, to help sweep out all the toxins you will be excreting.

- **TAKE ASHWAGANDHA.** Continue on the same dosage as Stage Two, but if you are still struggling with cravings, you can increase your dose to 800 to 1,000 milligrams, twice a day.

- **TAKE BRAHMI.** As with ashwagandha, continue as before, or increase your dose if you are still struggling with cravings and brain fog. You can take up to 1,000 milligrams, twice a day.

- **DRINK PRIME JUICE AND PRIME BROTH.** Continue to drink up to fight cravings and to supplement your nutritional status. If, in this stage, you start to experience more severe detox symptoms, increase the Prime Juice and Prime Broth to five days a week, if you aren't already there. You can also have them both twice a day. The more nutrition you add, the easier your detoxification will go.

- **JOURNAL YOUR CRAVINGS.** Continue to journal your cravings and if you like, add a note each day about how you are feeling, as your body goes deep and discards entrenched ama.

Guggul

Guggul is another of my secret weapons alongside triphala. It is the most powerful detoxifier I know, and when your body is ready for it, it can do incredible things. While you need triphala to support guggul's actions, guggul is the real superstar. Triphala prepares your body, and guggul is like an ama bulldozer.

Specifically, guggul boosts the detoxification power of the liver by increasing the quantity of cytochrome P450 enzymes in the liver and by upregulating the secretion of bile salts that specifically help remove fat from the liver.[1] This is the mechanism behind the ancient claim that guggul lowers blood cholesterol and fights obesity and heart disease. Many studies have noted powerful lipid-lowering effects from guggul.[2] In Ayurveda, it is said that guggul scrapes the ama out of the organs. This is a visual way of describing what studies show is the actual scientific mechanism behind its power: the way it increases those cytochrome P450 enzymes in the liver and makes the liver more efficient at removing toxins. Guggul also sends a signal to the organs to start mobilizing these toxins for removal. These include lipids in the arteries, which get flushed out through the liver. All the toxins that have accumulated deep in your tissues are getting pulled out now and being metabolized. Guggul is the reason why Stage Three is the most powerful detox stage of all (which you are only now prepared for, because you have worked through Stages One and Two).

Guggul is also excellent for helping your body respond appropriately to foods. For example, guggul ruined cheese for me. After I started taking it, I started noticing how hard cheese was on my digestive system. You may notice similar things—if the foods you ate before weren't making an impression on you, they definitely will once you start taking guggul. I used to love peanut butter chocolate ice cream, but after guggul, a couple of bites made me feel sick. It became so obvious to me what did not agree with my body. So many people eat and drink things that are having a bad effect on them, but they don't make the connection. "Why do I get headaches when I drink wine?" "Why do I get a stomachache when I have cheese?" "Why do I get heartburn every time I eat meat?" These are all signs of toxicity, and guggul helps you feel it keenly.

But don't worry—you won't feel the loss. When your dopamine begins to normalize, you will feel that food no longer has control over you. You aren't losing anything. The food is losing its control. The biggest shock is that you will stop thinking about those foods that used to rule you and your mind. You will stop thinking about cheese, ice cream, wine. It's pretty amazing.

If you look at the studies on guggul, you may notice that the dosages are higher than what I recommend here. Guggul is such a powerful detoxifier that I don't want to overwhelm you, even at this point in The Prime. I start you out with the lowest possible dosage that I know to be effective. You may find that you want to increase the dosage, after you adjust to Stage Three. As your detox symptoms get milder, you can begin to increase your dosage to 1,000 milligrams, twice a day. I wouldn't recommend going any higher than this unsupervised. Most people on The Prime will get good results on just 500 milligrams taken twice a day.

GUGGUL: CAUTION FOR PEOPLE ON BLOOD PRESSURE MEDICATION

Because guggul increases the rate of detoxification in the liver, it can also increase the rate of metabolism of blood pressure medication. The Prime, however, typically results in a blood pressure drop. This is one of the reasons why I don't want you to start with too much guggul too soon. If you are on blood pressure medication, this is a good time to get a medical evaluation of your condition. If your doctor can determine that your health condition is improving, this may be the time to get a thumbs-up for a reduction in dosage (or even, in some cases, elimination of medication; but please do not do this without your doctor's consent).

Prime Curry Powder

The next addition in Stage Three just happens to be incredibly tasty. And it's not just tasty, but it is key to igniting your agni, or digestive fire. This is crucial because as your detoxification ramps up, you need a strong digestive fire to help process all those toxins and get them out of your body. You can use this curry powder in any savory thing you are cooking (soup, sautéed vegetables, stir-fries, casseroles, etc.). You can also keep some in a saltshaker to sprinkle on your food whenever you want more flavor. Or, if you don't want to put it in your food, you can mix it into ½ cup of warm water and drink it before or after meals. If you tend to have problems with cravings and overeating, you can drink this concoction anywhere from twenty minutes before to just as you are about to eat a meal. If you tend to have more problems with digestion and absorption, getting bloated after meals, belching, having gas, and feeling sleepy after you eat, drink this after meals. Drink it quickly. It has a strong taste if it is not mixed with food, and it may be a little intense at first.

I like to make up a fresh batch every month. This recipe makes enough for about a month, depending on how liberally you use it. Aim for about ½ to 1 teaspoon per day in the beginning and then increase it to ½ to 1 teaspoon, twice a day.

Also note that you can grind the seeds that you are already using in your tea in a spice grinder for maximum freshness, but you can also buy ground seeds in powder form. You can find most of these ingredients at your grocery or health food store. If you are having trouble finding amla powder, look online or in an Indian grocery store. Prime Curry Powder has a delicious, savory taste that will give your meals an exotic flavor along with major health benefits. Here is how to make it:

Prime Curry Powder

8 teaspoons ground cumin seed (cumin powder)

8 teaspoons ground coriander seed (coriander powder)

8 teaspoons ground fennel seed (fennel powder)

8 teaspoons dried ginger powder (if you are sensitive to ginger, you can decrease this to 4 teaspoons, but I still advise including it, as it is quite beneficial)

4 teaspoons turmeric powder

4 teaspoons amla powder

Combine all the ingredients so they are well mixed together using a spoon and store in an airtight container. To use in cooking, add ½ teaspoon per serving. For example, if you were making a soup that served 8, you could add 4 teaspoons of this curry powder. (Adding more could overpower the food.)

I recommend that you cook with it. That makes it the most absorbable. It is important to have the taste of the spices in your mouth. A lot of the "miracle herbs" that come out are put in capsules. This is fine if the taste is so strong that people wouldn't tolerate them in powdered form. Prime Curry Powder is delicious, however, and adding it to food adds to its potency. It will have a greater impact on the brain and in coordinating the brain-gut relationship and the secretion of digestive enzymes because you can taste it.

Now let's talk about what is in this fantastic spice combination. You already learned what cumin, coriander, fennel, and amla berry powder do for you in Stage One. But what about the rest of the spices? How are ginger and turmeric powder helping you?

Ginger

Ginger is a flowering plant and its root (technically its rhizome) has been used for thousands of years in Indian cooking, and in many other cultures' cuisines as well. Ginger has a reputation for settling the stomach.[3] It has a calming effect on the GI tract and can decrease intestinal spasms and gas. Ginger is an excellent anti-inflammatory[4] because of compounds it contains called gingerols, and there is even some research suggesting it could have anticancer properties.[5] Another reason I like to introduce ginger in Stage Three is that it stimulates agni, the digestive fire. Ginger stimulates the release of digestive enzymes that increase the body's ability to break down food and absorb its nutrients.

Turmeric

Turmeric is related to ginger, and an extract of turmeric called curcumin is the part of this root that is most known for its health benefits. In India, turmeric is so common that most people eat it every day. There is a lot of evidence about the health benefits of turmeric. It has been shown to lower cholesterol, reduce blood sugar in people with blood sugar issues,[6] relieve arthritis pain,[7] reduce menstrual cramps, and reduce inflammation.[8] It may also speed wound healing and has been demonstrated to destroy many types of cancer cells.[9] Several studies have shown how curcumin can kill melanoma cells,[10] which tend to be resistant to chemotherapy, and colon cancer cells.[11] It has been shown to improve the symptoms of Alzheimer's disease.[12] I also find it extremely good for the skin. When I was growing up, turmeric made into a paste with a little water was a common remedy for any skin infection—it is antimicrobial, antiseptic, and anti-inflammatory. When we were sick, we would take a combination of turmeric and honey two or three times a day to treat most viral and bacterial infections in the upper respiratory system. It also makes a good face mask and can kill some of the bacteria associated with acne, but it has the most potent effect when you eat it. Its natural antimicrobial effect helps reestablish the good gut bacteria population and remove pathogens. As an anti-inflammatory, it helps heal the gut mucosa by reducing inflammation in the gut lining.

Ginger Gut Flush

The Ginger Gut Flush is one of the best ways I know to ignite agni, warm the body, and really power up digestive energy. I especially recommend the Ginger Gut Flush if you have more than thirty pounds to lose and/or if you scored in the medium to high range on the Gut IQ Test. I use it in the winter because that is when I notice a dip in my digestion and so its warming properties aid me in not accumulating ama. Here is how to make it:

Ginger Gut Flush

1 fresh lemon (or enough to make ½ cup juice)
1 inch peeled fresh ginger
½ teaspoon natural salt (preferably Himalayan salt or sea salt)

Squeeze the lemon to make ½ cup fresh lemon juice, strain out any seeds, and put the juice into a lidded jar. Cut the ginger into thin one-inch strips. Add these to the lemon juice. Add the salt to the mixture and stir until the salt dissolves. Cover and refrigerate.

Eat one to two pieces of the soaked fresh ginger before each meal. Make a batch at the beginning of the week and it will last for seven days in the refrigerator. If you want to slow down your detox symptoms, just eat it before your largest meal of the day, as opposed to before every meal. This will help your digestive fire get ready to digest your large meal but will put the brakes on too-fast detoxing.

Priming Your Body in Stage Three: How You Will Feel

You are going to experience a lot of changes in Stage Three. This is usually the stage with the greatest transformation because the guggul is pulling out such a deep level of toxins and you are increasing your agni, which begins to burn off all the old toxins physically, mentally, and emotionally. This is the stage where most people experience their greatest detox symptoms. It can feel intense. You may wonder why it takes so long to get to this stage, and if you've done seven-day or ten-day detoxes before and thought you "detoxed," this may seem strange to you. But there is a good reason why Stage Three is so intense. Shorter cleanses take care of the toxins on the "surface," which is important, but they don't even begin to address the toxins that have been held by the organs for so many years. Many of these toxins are lipophilic, or stored in fat—not just in your subcutaneous fat but also the fat in your organs. The guggul helps pull out long-term toxins that are often embedded within the fatty tissue of the organs. Shorter cleanses approximate some aspects of Stages One and Two of The Prime (although most are less thorough, in my experience). They help open up the colon and remove the surface waste in the GI tract, but you can't mobilize the deeper ama from the organs this way. But people usually stop there, and this is just the beginning. Stage Three is when things get really exciting—and possibly a little uncomfortable, temporarily. You may experience some of the following during Stage Three:

- Skin eruptions
- Headache
- Joint pain
- Nausea
- Loss of appetite (Pay attention to why! What are you eating that you don't really want now?)
- Thick, sticky, or strange-looking bowel movements, often of a higher volume than seems possible based on how much you are eating
- Fatigue or low energy
- Irritability
- Anxiety
- Depression
- Extremely vivid dreams
- Dissatisfaction with your job and/or relationships
- Questioning your life purpose

Trust me when I tell you that these uncomfortable symptoms will subside. For this reason, you should stay in this stage for as long as you need to and not rush to finish the program. Some of my patients stay at Stage Three for months.

Don't underestimate the emotional component of this stage. This is typically the most tumultuous part of The Prime because people begin to "wake up" to all the things that are out of balance in their lives—the way they eat, their job, their relationships. Your body and mind suddenly go into spring cleaning mode, and many people begin wanting to make changes in their lives. There tends to be a discomfort with where you currently are, but you don't have a sense yet of where you want to go or what to do about it. My advice is to not get overwhelmed. Don't feel you have to change everything at once.

That's not a recipe for success. Just start by paying attention to how your food makes you feel and make whatever changes feel spontaneous and easy. Then, as you have more body awareness, expand that awareness to how other aspects of your life make you feel and do the same thing—make the changes that feel spontaneous and easy. Taking small, consistent steps is a much more successful path to transformation than giant steps in every direction of your life.

STAGE THREE DETOX BOX

For a little extra help managing your detox symptoms in Stage Three, try the following:

1. More water, more tea, more fiber, more rest, more Prime Juice, and more Prime Broth—ramp up all those important first steps now.

2. You may need to increase your triphala dose if you begin to be constipated. Increase gradually, from 2,000 milligrams to 3,000 milligrams to a max of 4,000 milligrams, if needed. Stop at the level at which you are having a good bowel movement at least once per day.

3. Sweating more can help—use a sauna or Epsom salt baths on a weekly basis. (Don't worry about high-intensity exercise, especially during Stage Three. You are using a lot of energy for detoxification, so rerouting that energy for intense exercise can be counterproductive now.)

4. If your detox symptoms are really severe, back off on the guggul dose to only 500 milligrams daily. You can work back up as you get more comfortable.

5. If you are also working with a naturopathic doctor, functional medicine doctor, or other integrative practitioner, you may want to add supplements such as glutathione, alpha lipoic acid, and N-acetylcysteine to help manage the detoxification. *Only do this under medical supervision.*

How Long to Continue

Do not rush out of this stage. Instead, look for signs that the intensity is lessening, including the following:

- Detoxification symptoms becoming milder (they don't have to be completely gone)
- More energy and greater mental clarity and focus
- A feeling of calm and a reduction in anxiety and irritability

Once you feel these things, you can move on to Stage Four. If you are still detoxing considerably, however, it will be hard to make lifestyle changes. Be patient and stay here until you are in the clear. You can still have detox symptoms, but they should be manageable to the point that you are not struggling to get through the day. They too will soon subside as you work through Stage Four.

BIOHACK YOUR LIFESTYLE HABITS

You are probably feeling quite different than you did before you began The Prime. Perhaps you are more energetic. Your enteric nervous system is back online, and you have noticed that you have far fewer cravings than you did before. You've probably also lost some weight, maybe even a significant amount of weight, if you have weight to lose. This is all great, but we aren't finished yet. In this last stage of The Prime, we have some more important work to do, but it won't involve any additional spices, herbs, or adding anything else to your meals. Instead, we are going to concentrate on hacking your lifestyle to be more in line with your clean and vibrant body/mind.

This stage is largely about your schedule. Schedules tend to be habitual, and in this stage, you are going to shift some of your habits, forming new ones. This may feel intimidating at first because schedules can feel deeply ingrained. The fact that they are habits also means they can be changed. During this stage, for as long as you need to stay here, I want you to start shifting some things around, like mealtimes and bedtimes. You can do them all at once or one at a time. Remember, slower changes almost always make for more permanent changes, so don't be in a rush to finish this stage. Adjust slowly, gradually, and stay here until your new habits are ingrained, so that you would feel uncomfortable doing things the way you used to do them.

STAGE FOUR SNAPSHOT

- **EAT LARGEST AT LUNCH.** You will switch your largest meal to lunch and have a lighter dinner. You can still eat just as much; you're just shifting the time around.

- **WARM IT UP.** For now, raw food is off the menu. All your food and drinks should be warm—not just your tea but your water, that ice-cold glass of lemonade you were thinking about having, even your salad. You can toss a salad in a warm skillet for a minute or two before eating it. All this will make everything you put in your mouth more digestible.

- **MEDITATE.** It's easy and it will change your life. You just have to make a small space for it in your schedule.

- **EARLY TO BED.** Your new bedtime is 10 p.m. If you usually stay up much later, it's time to start downshifting. Move your bedtime up by fifteen to thirty minutes each week until you are turning the lights off at 10:00.

Continue These Healthy Habits:

- **GUGGUL.** Continue to take 500 milligrams twice a day, or a higher dose if you were able to increase it during Stage Three.

- **PRIME CURRY POWDER.** Continue to take 1/2 to 1 teaspoon per day with meals, or more if you increased the amount in Stage Three.

- **GINGER GUT FLUSH.** Continue to take two to three pieces per day with lunch and/or dinner.

- **ASHWAGANDHA.** Continue to take 400 to 500 milligrams twice per day, or whatever dose you were taking in Stage Three.

- **BRAHMI.** Continue to take 400 to 500 milligrams twice per day, or whatever dose you were taking in Stage Three.

- **NOURISH WITH PRIME JUICE AND PRIME BROTH.** Continue to enjoy these as needed.

- **JOURNAL YOUR CRAVINGS.** Continue to journal your cravings. You will have many opportunities for exploring and tuning into your self-awareness in Stage Four.

- **DRY-BRUSH YOUR SKIN** before your morning shower using a raw silk glove or an actual brush designed for dry-brushing.

- **DRINK YOUR PRIME TEA,** and sip on it throughout the day, as before.

- **TAKE TRIPHALA,** 1,000 milligrams per day or your previous dosage.

- **TAKE FIBER,** 1 teaspoon per day or your previous dosage.

You may already be thinking that you can do some of these life-style hacks, but you don't think you can do all of them. Maybe you can't possibly eat your largest meal at lunch (or so you think), or it would be inconceivable to go to bed by 10 p.m. But bear with me. Let's look at the reasons why these changes are so important, and why they not only are possible for you but can be the final nail in the coffin of your former health-wrecking habits.

All About Lunch

In U.S. culture, it is traditional to eat the largest meal in the evening, but this is much harder on your digestion than eating the bulk of your calories during the middle of the day, when you most require energy. This is an ancient Ayurvedic concept, but it is practiced in many other cultures as well (such as in Europe). There is some research to back this up, too, such as one study that showed that eating out of sync with your circadian rhythm, which uses more energy during the day and less energy at night, can lead to insulin resistance, obesity, and type 2 diabetes.[1] Another study showed that eating a larger breakfast and lunch and skipping or having a small dinner resulted in more weight loss and better blood sugar control than eating six small meals during the day.[2]

In Ayurveda, your agni (digestive fire) is linked to the cycles of the sun. When the sun is the strongest (at noon), that is also when your agni is the strongest in your body. Eating more at lunchtime is simply more efficient—you absorb more nutrients and create less ama when your body is running at full steam. I always have a big lunch and if I'm going to have a heavy food or a dessert, I try to have it at lunchtime. Dinnertime is when your body begins to prepare for detoxification, which predominantly occurs during the night when your body is at rest. (This is also why most people have a bowel movement in the morning—the body is expelling the waste it was processing while you slept.) If you have a large dinner, not only does it tend to disrupt sleep, but it also makes detoxification less effective because your body has to expend extra energy breaking down the food you consumed at dinner.

Some people complain that they get tired after they eat, which is why they don't want to eat a large lunch. They want to wait until the end of the day when they don't need any more energy. If you get tired after eating, though, it's due to weak digestion. This should already be correcting itself based on what you've been doing during the first three stages. You are probably now hungrier during the day and less hungry at night, as you become more attuned to your body's natural rhythms.

Still, culture is a strong influence. You may think (especially if you are reading this before you've started Stage Three) that this will be impossible to do. Your family likes to have a big dinner together at night! You like to go out with your friends and eat a lot and drink wine! I understand this. I used to be a big dinner socializer. Logically, I would tell myself that I could still socialize at dinner without eating a lot, but when everyone else was eating, I felt left out if I wasn't eating, too.

As I said before, though, this is really just a habit and changing it is easier than you think. (And you don't have to quit socializing!) After taking the guggul, it becomes really hard to do things that harm your body, just for the sake of socializing. Guggul helps you *feel* when you should eat more, and when you should eat less. If you overdo dinner, the social part will feel less fun because you are making yourself sick each time you go against your body, and you feel it acutely.

It's not just a theory about "eating a big lunch and a light dinner" anymore. It's real in your body. The overactivation of the dopamine system adds to the social "high" of eating out, but when that normalizes, the food is really a minor part of the evening and your friends become the highlight.

Also, as you work through Stage Three, you will find that eating a light dinner is a much smaller "sacrifice" than you thought it would be. (My definition of a light dinner is eating about half what you eat at lunch, with more vegetables and soupy foods and less high-fat food and meat that requires a lot of digestive energy.) You are more in touch with your "internal family" (your organs) now, and you realize the price you pay each time you harm them. I no longer enjoy eating a big dinner, but that doesn't mean I can't sit down with family or friends for an evening meal. We used to go out with friends for dinner a few times every week. Now I shudder at the thought because if I do this and eat too much, I am sick for a few days afterward. If I go out with friends now, we go out for lunch. Or, if dinner plans are inevitable, I order light food and focus on the company and the conversation. I am not there to overeat. I am there to enjoy the people I'm with. Also, as my health habits have changed, my social circle has changed and no one I socialize with regularly finds big dinners that enjoyable anymore. Even my family members, who I thought would never adapt, eventually changed when they developed health problems and realized that they felt better eating less in the evening, too.

The problem is not that you will be missing out on the socialization at dinner; the problem is that up until now your ENS has not been up and running properly. Until it comes online, these things feel like hard choices. Once it's in charge, you wonder how on earth you lived any other way. That is why I don't recommend people try to do this step until after they have started the guggul. Many of my patients are initially the only ones in their families making healthy choices, but for them it is no longer a choice—they just can't feel sick and tired all the time. Sometimes it takes their family members two to three years to catch on and sometimes they never do, but for my patients, it becomes easy to stick to their habits. The benefits outweigh the temporary dopamine highs once your ENS is at the helm, so that living this way feels not just worthwhile but inevitable. It's really a chemical switch that gets flipped—not a mental one—and once it is switched, the healthy habits are pretty spontaneous.

WHAT ABOUT BREAKFAST?

A lot of my patients ask me what to do about breakfast when they are shifting their largest meal to lunch. This really depends on your agni and how you feel in the morning. My digestion is not strong enough to make me crave breakfast. I tend to have some warm water with lemon when I wake up, and maybe some warm milk for breakfast, but I don't usually eat anything until about 10 a.m., when I have a small snack, like some almonds or dried fruit. Then I have a huge lunch because I'm usually really hungry around noon. Dinner is small, often just some soup or grilled vegetables.

However, sometimes when I am getting more physical exercise, I am hungrier in the morning, and then I have breakfast. See how you feel in the morning. If you are hungry, have breakfast, keeping in mind that you will be eating a big lunch. If you aren't hungry, don't force yourself to have it. Everyone is different. You may typically be a breakfast eater, or you may not be. Pay attention to how you feel, especially after you have had a big lunch for a few days. You may find that your desire for breakfast decreases or perhaps increases. Either way, respect your body's cues. Trust your body instincts.

No-Raw Zone

The next important lifestyle hack may sound strange to you: I don't want you to eat any raw vegetables. You can eat raw fruit (except for apples, which should be cooked), but other than that, all the solid food you eat should be cooked. This may seem counterintuitive. Isn't a raw diet the way to lose weight? And don't we need more salads on a diet? Actually, no. Cooking food here is about two things:

1. Warming it to increase blood flow to your gut and improve digestion
2. Making it easier to digest by breaking down some of the cellular matrices so that nutrients are more bio-available.

There is research to support this. One study analyzed the effect of cooking on nutrient availability in vegetables and found that cooking in water (such as steaming or boiling) better preserved antioxidant content, especially of carotenoids but also of vitamin C. Also, antioxidant capacity was improved in all cooking methods. The study surmised that this was "because of matrix softening and increased extractability of compounds."[3]

Beyond nutrition, however, raw vegetables can simply be hard to digest. Anybody with irritable bowel syndrome knows this. You can chew and chew but cold hard raw food can upset the digestion, especially when it isn't working at optimum capacity. When you are fully Primed, you can eat your big salad at lunchtime (I never recommend raw food at dinner because of lower agni at night), but for now, hold off on that and opt for cooked veggies instead. Steam them, sauté them, or poach them, but give your digestion that extra boost. Cooking them in ghee (clarified butter) makes them even more digestible because ghee increases agni. (I'll talk more about ghee in the next chapter.)

As for beverages, I told you about the benefits of warm drinks when I gave you the recipe for Prime Tea. Starting now, this should apply to all your beverages. Just say no to ice. Drink your water warm or at room temperature, and avoid chilled beverages of all kinds. No ice-cold lemonade, no ice-cold beer, no ice-cold soda, and no ice water. If room-temperature water and herbal teas are your beverages of choice, your digestion will run more smoothly. If you have traveled outside the United States, you've noticed that most other cultures never put ice in their beverages. Now you know the reason why.

Daily Brain Detox: Meditation

Although I was tempted to introduce it earlier in the program, I have waited until now to add meditation to the plan, because I want to be sure you are ready for it. Meditation is potent medicine for the brain. It is also a necessary component of mental detoxing. I often talk to my patients about how emotions will begin to come out, like mental toxins, as the body releases deeper levels of physical toxins. Now that you have completed Stage Three and you have been taking guggul, you may have noticed that your emotions are in upheaval. Maybe you are having mood swings: bouts of joy and sudden crashes of sadness. Maybe you are more irritable than usual or you feel angry without knowing why. Remember that depression, when it starts to release in the body, often becomes anger, which is where it started. This means your toxic emotions are coming out, and that's great, but without a strategy to deal with them, you are at risk of becoming overwhelmed and even quitting the program. Emotions are powerful. But so is meditation.

But meditation does more than help you deal with emotions. It also has a direct anti-inflammatory effect on the brain and body. Meditation reverses the whole stress response and its cascade of signals,[4] and it improves immune function.[5] It has even been used successfully to treat chronic pain.[6] It regulates the way the brain fires, making your central nervous system smarter and improving the brain-gut connection. Several studies show how meditation reduces the severity of gut-related dysfunction, such as digestive issues[7] and irritable bowel syndrome.[8] Meditation is great for your brain. It improves attention and self-control[9] and is an effective treatment for anxiety disorders[10] and attention deficit/hyperactivity disorder (ADHD) in both adults and children.[11] Meditation is particularly good for getting back in control of cravings. As you now know, cravings are caused by overstimulation of the pleasure centers, leading to neuroadaptation and addiction, but meditation blocks that overstimulation response, teaching the brain not to be fooled by it. Studies have demonstrated a reduction in substance abuse with meditation.[12] Meditation also naturally and gently increases serotonin, so you feel good even in the face of detox symptoms. Hundreds of studies demonstrate these effects. It is indisputably a beneficial practice. Its benefits are so powerful and pervasive that I recommend meditation as a new habit for a lifetime.

But how do you do it? I was trained in Transcendental Meditation (TM), one of the most widely studied forms of meditation, originating in India. I find TM extremely easy and highly beneficial. It works for me, and it is the form of meditation that I recommend to my patients. TM is a form of mantra meditation, meaning you repeat a sound in your mind using special techniques that require an instructor, who assures you are doing it correctly. You can take a course to learn TM, which I recommend, or you can try other techniques if you prefer. Many of these are explained in books, in apps, on websites, and even on videos or CDs that guide you through the meditation technique. Studies show benefits from many different types of meditation (although TM usually comes out on top). Simply sitting quietly without distractions and focusing on your breathing for fifteen to twenty minutes once or twice a day will have noticeable benefits. The most important thing is to find a meditation practice that fits you and start doing it regularly.

Early to Bed

Finally, I want you to go to bed by 10 p.m. This may be earlier than you are used to going to sleep, but this is one of the best things you can do for your health. For the same reasons I want you to eat your biggest meal at noon, I want you to go to bed before 10 p.m. This is how to take best advantage of your natural circadian rhythms. Detoxification energy rises in the body at 10 p.m. If you happen to be awake after 10 p.m., you will hit your second wind. This then turns into mental energy and you may find that suddenly you can't fall asleep and may lie awake for two hours. You may find you get hungry at midnight. That's because in being awake you have misdirected the energy that was meant for detoxification. Between 10 p.m. and 2 a.m., you should be getting your most restful, deep, and regenerative sleep.

Going to bed earlier is also important to avoid sleep deprivation, since most people have to get up by a certain time. One good reason to turn in earlier is that two hormones that regulate your appetite—a hormone called ghrelin, which signals to you that you are hungry and need to eat, and a hormone called leptin, which signals to you that you are full and should stop eating—get dis-regulated in people who are sleep-deprived. This is why people who don't get enough sleep tend to be hungrier and overeat, especially sugars, and tend to weigh more.[13] Sleep is an important investment in your health, even if it means you have to record your favorite late-night show and watch it in the early evening.

On The Prime, chances are good that you are already feeling more sensitive to your body's natural rhythms and desiring an earlier bedtime. Please heed this biological call, as it is extremely important for detoxification. If you absolutely cannot do this because of your job, then at least get sufficient sleep (about eight hours per night) and be vigilant about all the other detoxification protocols.

Priming Your Body in Stage Four: How You Will Feel

This is typically the stage where things really start coming together. People feel better in significant ways, and these habits in particular help "seal" their new biochemistry into their lives. After implementing the suggestions in Stage Four, people feel more balanced. They feel like they are walking out of a prison. Their moods are more stable, their energy is higher, and they experience more mental clarity, significantly fewer cravings, and of course weight loss. But most importantly, people feel armed to begin tackling all the changes that they are now seeing they want to make in life. It feels less daunting and there is a newfound confidence because now there is a set of tools to approach challenges in a new way. Challenges are a part of life, but now you're Primed to face them.

How Long to Continue

When you feel like you have fully tackled your cravings, your moods are stable, your brain is clear, and you have lost the weight you want to lose, you are ready to move on and maintain The Prime.

CHAPTER 7

LIVING PRIMED

Once you have made your way through all four stages, it is time to decide when you are fully Primed. How do you know you have achieved this? The most important sign that you are ready to move on to a maintenance program is that your mind and body know what you need to do to feel good and be healthy. You are in touch with yourself on a daily basis. You can feel whether a choice you make is right for your mind and body.

At this point, I would like you to retake the Gut IQ Test on page 118. This will give you a good indication of the progress you have made, and it will also let you know how far you still have to go. Your new Gut IQ score can tell you that you aren't quite done with Stage Four yet and you should stay the course, or it may look pretty good, meaning you can proceed to a maintenance version of The Prime.

Once you do that, the first thing to do is decide which parts of The Prime you want to keep for yourself, for the rest of your life. This differs according to the individual, as different people respond more favorably to different parts. For example, you could never convince me to give up triphala, psyllium husks, or Prime Tea, because they make me feel so good. My body responds in a positive way and I can feel it, so that is the only motivation I need to keep those things in my life. You no longer have to convince me that lassi (a diluted yogurt drink) with my lunch is a good thing because when I drink it, I don't feel that midafternoon decline. (I'll tell you more about lassi a little later.) If I miss my morning meditation, I feel it all day. I get a stress response to missing my meditation because I have neuroadapted to the peaceful state I achieve from meditation. When I'm stressed out, my family knows to give me time, to let me go meditate, because that solves the problem so quickly and easily. Sometimes I know I have to do it right at that moment. It can't wait. You can't even ask me one question. I have to go do it now! Positive neuroadaptation makes you crave, require, and be "addicted" to habits that keep you healthier, feeling better, thinking clearer, and at a normal body weight.

Next, consider what your habits are right now. You know you are Primed when you have neuroadapted to positive behaviors, and your ENS (rather than bad gut bacteria) is making decisions about what to eat. When you are in a positive feedback loop instead of a negative feedback loop, you will know what you need. You will know when you need that time-out or that bone broth or that you need to go to bed now. This is how you take care of yourself. This is how you live.

When all four stages have done their work and you are neuro-adapted to those new behaviors, you can switch into a maintenance routine that you can practice most of the time. When an event comes up, when you travel, or just because it's the weekend, you can now indulge in the occasional decadent treat without ruining your progress because your body is Primed to handle it. On most days, however, I suggest integrating these Prime habits into your new life. They should already be easy because you've been doing them for so long now.

Daily Maintenance Habits

You can adjust these to your preference, but in general, these are my recommendations for daily health maintenance:

- If you have increased your dosage of triphala, you can bring it back down now, but continue to take it daily. I typically recommend that you take from 1,000 milligrams to no more than 2,000 milligrams every evening.

- You don't have to take the fiber quite so often if your digestion is working. I recommend the psyllium husks and flax seeds about twice a week. If you notice that your digestion is getting sluggish, add more fiber until things start to move along smoothly again.

- Many of my patients continue with Prime Tea because they have grown so accustomed to it. Typically, I recommend continuing to drink the tea on weekdays, Monday through Friday, but you can take a break on the weekends. You can also adjust your Prime Tea consumption seasonally. Your body needs a little more help with digestion and warmth in the fall and winter if you are eating heavy foods and you live in a cold climate. I suggest drinking the tea Monday through Friday during the fall and winter, but cutting back to two or three days per week during the spring and summer. I have it about twice a week, but when I'm traveling or doing anything stressful, or if I get sick or the weather gets really cold, I'll increase it to five days per week or more.

- For most of my patients, I recommend that they continue to take the ashwagandha and Brahmi every day. These are neuroregenerative herbs that can be taken on a regular basis with no negative effects, and they confer such strong brain benefits as you age that I think everyone will feel better taking them. If you have increased your dose, you could decrease your dose back down to 400 to 500 milligrams twice a day of each. This is a good maintenance dose.

- I suggest continuing to cook with the Prime Curry Powder as often as you can. Daily is not too often. Sometimes I also mix a teaspoon into warm water when my digestion feels off or I feel like I need to stoke my agni.

- Meditation is an essential part of my life and I have nothing but good things to say about it. If you can continue to do it once or preferably twice every day for the rest of your life, you will enjoy major benefits in both body and mind.

- Whenever you can, continue with your lifestyle hacks: eat your largest meal at lunch most of the time and go to bed by 10 p.m. on most nights. The more you do this, the easier it gets. I recognize that our culture is designed around light lunches and large dinners, but if you can eat light in the evening and get to bed earlier, you will feel lighter, stronger, and more energetic, and you will have beaten one of our culture's worst habits.

Seasonal or As-Needed Remedies

These habits aren't necessarily for every day. Because you are more body-aware now, you should be able to cue in to when your body needs these special digestive and nutrient boosters.

- I suggest taking guggul seasonally. Bring it back into your life in early fall for one month, and then in early spring for one month. These are ideal cleansing times when your body is shifting into a new mode, and guggul will help with that transition by invoking a deep cleaning. It's like spring cleaning (and fall cleaning) your entire digestive system. Spring in particular is a time when your liver naturally begins to detox, so adding guggul at this time gives you the most bang for your buck. Recently, I've also started to use a little guggul during the holidays, which is a time when many people get derailed from healthy habits, because it keeps my holiday eating in check.

- I also recommend the Ginger Gut Flush seasonally. Make up batches during the fall or winter, or whenever you feel like your digestion is slowing down. I particularly like it in the fall because that's when my digestion tends to go off track.

- You can always enjoy Prime Broth and Prime Juice, but you don't have to have them constantly if you don't want to. But keep them in your rotation if you like them and they make you feel good. They are also good to add back in when you are bringing guggul back in seasonally, as indicated earlier. Or bring them back onto the menu when you're not getting a lot of concentrated nutrition, such as when you're traveling or working longer hours. There is certainly no downside.

- Whenever your digestion feels weak (you are getting indigestion, gas, bloating) or you feel fatigued or mentally foggy, lack creativity, or start gaining weight, go back to the ban on raw foods and cold beverages. Cook most of your food (except for fruits, other than apples) and avoid cold beverages until things feel right again. This is particularly likely to happen in the fall and winter, when your body may struggle to stay warm and your digestion may stall again. If you decide never to go back to cold beverages again, that is perfectly fine.

When to Repeat The Prime

Because The Prime is such an effective detox, I recommend doing it twice a year, during nature's seasonal cleansing times when the body naturally lapses into a detoxification pattern: fall and spring. You don't have to spend as long at each stage when you repeat The Prime. If you are feeling good, a week for each stage should be enough to get you ready for the next season. If you've lapsed into bad habits and you are feeling like you need more cleansing, spend longer. There is never any reason to rush. Health is a journey and The Prime is your vehicle. Relax, rejuvenate, and take care of yourself, and everything about your life will feel better.

I am pretty strict about the way I live now because I've gotten "addicted" to feeling good and I follow many of the principles I will introduce to you in the next few chapters, but those changes of seasons become obvious in the body even for me. The Prime is body-led maintenance, so pay attention to how you feel and act accordingly. My goal for you is to get you to the point where you can feel when you need to do certain things because you know how they help you. This isn't an overnight process. True body understanding takes practice. With persistence, my patients get there, and you can, too.

The Middle Way

Finally, I want to emphasize one thing: It is never good to be overly rigid. When I first became vegetarian, then vegan, I was really rigid about it. I ate nothing from animals, but it didn't take me long to notice that this wasn't good for my body. It took a lot of convincing for me to do the bone broth, and then to reincorporate ghee and lassi into my diet, but these changes worked well for me. I still consider myself mostly vegan because I believe (and research supports) that this is the healthiest (and most humane and most environmentally respectful) way to eat.

When you are extremely rigid, there is a point of diminishing returns. You lose flexibility in your mind and in your body. On the other hand, I have also gone through extremely lax phases when I lapsed into bad habits that also caused me harm I could feel. There is a happy medium, and each one of us must find it for ourselves. In my family, one day a week, our child gets to choose where we eat and we have fun with it. Occasionally, I indulge in sweets, which are considered medicinal in certain forms and in small amounts in Ayurvedic medicine. I stay away from processed foods most of the time, but I try to keep it relaxed and walk the middle path. This helps balance the mind as well as the body, and when your body and mind are Primed, they can handle it.

You've done it. You've completed The Prime, and the best news about that is your new life is just beginning. Now you can accomplish lifestyle changes you couldn't accomplish before. You've probably already done some of that spontaneously, but there are more to come! In the next section of the book, I have even more information for you—information about how to live and thrive when you are Primed.

PART FOUR

Secrets of the Super-Primed

CHAPTER 8

ANCIENT FOOD KNOWLEDGE FOR THE MODERN WORLD

I haven't mentioned food much yet because until you were Primed, you weren't ready to change. You weren't ready to force yourself to give up the foods that your brain and gut were addicted to. I didn't want you to focus on what you were choosing to eat, beyond paying attention to how your body responded to foods as you began the detoxification and digestive healing process. This must come first. Without managing the toxic inflammatory state, your attempts to change your diet will likely be temporary and unsuccessful.

But now all that has changed. Now you are ready, so let's finally talk seriously about that thing you do three or more times every day: Eat.

What Are You Eating?

Now that you have completed The Prime, your food choices have probably changed spontaneously, maybe even significantly. But maybe they haven't changed as much as you would like, or maybe you are inspired to go even further. Food choices are an excellent way to further refine your health and continue your progress.

So what should you eat? People are more educated than ever before about nutrition because this information is so widely available, but at the same time, they are also more confused than ever. When you read about and hear about multiple food perspectives, and they all make sense in a way, it can be difficult to understand what you should do. The result is that many people become afraid to eat anything; or they do the reverse and eat everything while throwing their hands up in surrender.

This is a valid fear when it comes to processed and refined foods because these definitely contribute to a toxic inflammatory state due to the high load of "new-to-nature" chemicals and altered substances they contain. The fear goes beyond this, however. Many of my patients are terrified of carbs or fearful of fat or have a love-hate relationship with sugar. This can happen after years of indoctrination by various fad diets.

Being afraid of your food misses the point, though. The real point is that if you strengthen your digestion, your body as a whole becomes less vulnerable to the potentially deleterious effects of foods like grains, fat, and sugar when eaten with a weak digestive system. Processed, new-to-nature foods are never health-enhancing, but whole-food versions of grains, fats, and sugars can be good for you, and a strong digestion can tolerate the occasional fake food without much physical stress or trouble. In fact, there is a central theme in Ayurvedic medicine: if you have strong digestion, you can even eat poison; but if you have weak digestion, even the healthiest foods turn into poison.

Obviously you don't want to go out and eat poison! But "poison" is how many now see carbs or fat or sugar, not just because they have been told they are bad, but because they legitimately feel bad when they eat them. Even people who fastidiously avoid so-called bad foods often don't feel well, and they don't understand why. I see this over and over again. As my own medical practice has attracted an increasing number of health-conscious people, the complaint I often get when they first come to see me is, "I'm eating all the right things and I still don't feel healthy," or "I don't have any chronic disease according to my doctors, so why don't I feel good?"

Some of these people have had a chronic disease and have recovered through severe dietary restriction and other practices, but given the amount of work they are doing being so selective with the foods they are eating, they still feel like they are barely surviving. It's true: at any given moment, this precarious sort of state—dietary rigidity without the benefit of energy or vitality—could turn into a disease state again. It's a fragile feeling of health and only present under the most pristine conditions. To me, this is still imprisonment, even though it's a better prison than the prison of addiction and disease. It's like going from some terrible dirty solitary confinement cell into that prison Martha Stewart was in. But it's still a prison.

The reason that dietary restriction alone may help you find a precarious balance that can't technically be categorized as disease but does not have a firm health foundation is, again, digestion. If your digestion is strong, you will feel strong, vital, and energetic, and you won't have to live in a food prison. You won't have to be quite so careful about carbs or fat or unrefined sugar or anything else you love but think you can't have, especially if you indulge in the healthier versions of these foods (whole grains such as brown rice, unrefined fats such as those in avocadoes or ghee, and natural sugars such as coconut palm sugar and real maple syrup).

With a strong digestion, you can still have your favorite foods in moderation. If they are rich, pleasurable, and caloric foods, healthy digestion will tell your brain that you don't need them all the time. By healthy digestion, you now know I mean neuroadaptation to nutrient-rich foods, an appropriately penetrable gut and brain, a balanced gut flora, and a strong and online ENS. These send the clear message that the foods you love can be part of your life as treats that enrich your experience on special occasions, rather than dictators that rule your daily life.

The whole purpose of The Prime is to free you from *all prisons*—the prison of disease and dysfunction, and the prison of severe dietary restriction. My goal for you is that you live in a way that healthy habits create pleasure for you and you follow them be-cause you *want to*, because it feels right and good for you to do so, rather than because you *have to*, because it feels punitive or like a threat ("Eat this or else!"). I want your strong digestive system to allow you to thrive even when you don't have every possible good option in front of you. I want you to have *digestive resilience*. That doesn't mean you should be eating "poisons" such as toxic, pro-cessed foods on a regular basis, but if it happens once in a while, digestive resilience will allow you to bounce back without Hercu-lean efforts.

But healing takes time. In some people, it happens quickly. Their digestion may be strong and sound by the end of Stage Four. For oth-ers, however, it can take longer. The time it takes to heal depends on the extent of the damage. However, after the four stages, my pa-tients tend to be ready and asking for nutritional information. They can sense that they are ready to make some lifestyle changes—that these changes will feel easier and more natural. They want to know how to eat in a way that will not further aggravate any problems and slow down progress but will still be pleasurable and interesting. They are becoming more aware that some of their favorite foods now make them feel awful. Yet they don't want to have to learn by trial and error alone. They crave this information at this point in the journey, so this is the part of the book where I provide it for you. To break it down:

1. You should be able to eat just about any natural, whole food and feel good most of the time. *But . . .*

2. Many people can't eat even healthy foods without feeling poorly.

So where is the disconnect? You've already overcome some of it. The Prime has helped your body become more sensitive to those foods that are not healing as well as those that make you feel good, and your digestion is now stronger than it was before. But you may still feel compelled to practice some form of dietary restriction, or you may be compelled to rebel against any restrictions at all. Now that you are really thinking about food, you may be confused about what to do, exactly.

Fear not. The Prime will eventually help you come to the information and conclusions in this chapter on your own. The reality is that even if people just continued to do the maintenance part of The Prime, they would and will make a lot of the changes I'll suggest in this chapter spontaneously, gently, over the course of three to five years. You have probably already made some of them before you even began reading this chapter.

But if you feel ready for more change, you don't have to wait three to five years. I'm going to save you some time. Now that you are biochemically prepared to make some dietary changes, this chapter contains my guidance. Remember that changing your diet was not necessary for the initial healing and initial weight loss. Now that you have achieved this, you can take your health—physical and mental, body and brain—to the next level, if that is your desire.

Eat Whole Food

Let's start with a basic premise, and some basic advice that may or may not be obvious to you. Not so long ago, whole food was the only kind of food available. It is only recently (in the scope of human history) that processed, packaged, and highly refined foods have been not just available but preferred by most people. They say you can't stop progress, but this is one area where "progress" has hurt us. Food contains information for your body. The complexity and completeness of whole food is "educational" to your biochemistry. It helps support a smart gut by teaching it all the right things. Processed and artificial foods, however, offer incomplete, altered, or false information to the gut. It's like receiving a subpar or misleading education. Whereas whole food is the dynamic, brilliant professor who shares lessons that serve as tools for your life, processed/

artificial foods are the dull, boring, uninterested teacher who is phoning it in, whose attitude and false information can mislead you and slow your progress in life.

Unfortunately, we've gotten so far away from what food is supposed to look and taste like that we've forgotten all it can be— we are so used to the bad teachers that we don't recognize they are bad anymore. We think they are "normal." The information I would like you to reclaim, your right as a human designed to eat whole food, is just this: that food in its natural form, as it would look if picked from a stalk or pulled from the ground or plucked from a tree (or possibly hunted) is safe to eat and not an enemy to your body.

Whole food does not (for the most part) come from a can or a bag or a box. It is food without added preservatives, chemicals, artificial colors or flavors, or even added salt, sugar, or fat. It is fresh (like blueberries or a stalk of asparagus) and it contains all its original parts (like brown rice) rather than having its original parts removed (as in white flour). Once you have the whole food, you can certainly do things to it—cook it, bake it, stew it, or throw it into a soup. It still counts.

But what do most people eat today, in the modern world? Convenience food. This happened gradually—first, food was partially cooked and canned or frozen for us (something we used to do for ourselves). Then it was flavored and preserved and put on a shelf. It was fractionated and injected with chemicals to keep it looking and tasting like food. Finally, it was changed until you couldn't even recognize a whole food in what you unwrap, unpack, or microwave.

Can we get back to the diet we are designed to eat? Of course we can, but it's not always as easy as it would seem. Convenience is a powerful motivator in our fast-paced world. For some people, eating whole foods is a huge shift. For others, it's not a foreign concept; they just need to increase the amount of it in their diet.

But like everything else, I want to encourage you to go slow. I want to make it clear that when I tell you to eat whole food, I am not telling you that you have to change over to 100 percent whole food overnight. People who are used to convenience food can get overwhelmed by the idea of eating all whole food. They aren't always sure what it is (is brown rice a whole food since it comes in a bag?) or how to cook it. What I recommend is taking steps in the right direction. It's a transition.

Start by choosing one or two foods each day that look like they could have been picked from a garden or an orchard: a pear when you might have chosen a cookie, perhaps, or fresh steamed green beans instead of frozen, flavored green beans in sauce. It took me a couple of years to really embrace this concept, so why should it take you any less time? It isn't always easy or possible to eat whole foods at every single meal. If you eat whole foods *most of the time*, though, you will find that they provide you with the greatest possible nutrient density, feeding your body with what it needs.

VEGETARIANS BEWARE!

You may feel like a virtuous vegetarian eating your veggie burgers and veggie hot dogs, but if you are seeking better health through whole foods, be aware that a lot of these products are highly processed soy and are not whole foods. There are some good brands out there, made from whole grains, beans, and veggies, but most of the "veggie meats" are highly processed soy products. You are better off preparing simple vegetarian fare yourself. A sautéed slice of fresh tofu or tempeh is a better option than a processed veggie burger or dog.

Choose the Right Grains

There is a lot of press lately about the so-called dangers of grains. I have found that there is a lot of confusion about grains, especially with the popularity of the low-carb and paleo-style diets. A lot of dieters now believe that grains are bad for everyone, across the board.

There are some strong arguments about the deleterious effects of excessive carbohydrates. I tend to be skeptical, however, about any unilateral argument that an entire whole food group is bad for all people. This doesn't allow for biological diversity. "Grains are bad" is not an Ayurvedic perspective at all. Too much of anything can be harmful to the body, and people do tend to overeat grains in America, but the grains themselves are not the problem. In Ayurvedic medicine, grains are considered very nourishing, but they are also considered "rich" foods that should be consumed in accordance with the strength of your agni and your body type.

As you get older, your digestion naturally gets weaker. In general, I recommend fewer carbohydrates, especially less sugar, as people get older, in order to maintain a healthy microbiome and to reduce energy input as exercise and muscle mass may be decreasing. For most people, though, growing older means the body changes in certain ways—becoming thinner and smaller—that can benefit from small quantities of grains, for strength and substance.

But things have changed in our culture. People in America are becoming obese as they age, which is totally unnatural—and grains aggravate this condition. We do not digest grains as well because of increasing imbalances and digestive disturbances associated with abnormal weight gain together with aging. That's why we are seeing so many problems with grains, and so many people claiming to have grain sensitivities. Again, grains *should be nourishing* as you age, but eaten in smaller quantities because your overall food intake should naturally be less as you get older. But instead, grains have become toxic for those who are aging and simultaneously gaining unhealthy weight and body mass.

So what do we do about this problem? Do we swear off grains for good? No. Instead, we have to heal the digestion and balance the system so that you can benefit from grains the way you are meant to benefit. As you work with your diet and your digestion and as you get solid on maintenance with The Prime, a good rule of thumb is to make your proportion of vegetables at any given meal significantly higher than your proportion of grains. When agni is low (digestion is weak), we typically recommend only the most digestible grains, such as white, aged basmati rice. If you are having digestive issues with grains, gently refined natural ones may be easier for you, until your digestion is stronger. Brown rice has more nutrients than white basmati rice, but if you can't break it down, those nutrients won't do you any good. They will just turn toxic in your gut, transforming into ama. What is nutritious *for you* depends on what your gut can digest.

Those who have unstable blood sugar, inflammation, and insulin resistance must also be more careful with all carbohydrate sources until this instability is resolved. In general, for weight loss and with aging, a high-grain diet is not recommended. As people get older, their digestion naturally gets a little weaker. That means naturally, you should be inclined to eat less overall, in the absence of preexisting food addictions. If you remain healthy with a strong agni as you age, grains are nourishing and fortifying and can be a daily part of your diet in moderation without a problem.

Once your digestion is repaired, whole grains can be a staple of your diet, especially if you are not a meat eater and grains agree with you (and your newly repaired gut). Think about how many cultures on the planet survive on carbohydrate-rich food, whether rice or starchy tubers. Billions of people eat like this and are perfectly healthy. We don't see the kinds of health consequences in these people, who are eating natural diets, that we see in the United States. I believe this is because we eat way too much processed grain and refined sugar, and that has compromised our gut integrity and digestive health. In excess, grains and sugar are inflammatory, especially when they are processed. They can contribute to leaky gut and leaky brain. In moderation, in a healthy gut, they are usually just fine in combination with a whole-foods diet.

WHOLE VS. REFINED

A whole grain has had no part of the grain removed (such as the bran or germ) and has nothing added (such as flavoring). Examples include brown rice, quinoa, oats, millet, teff, buckwheat, spelt, and amaranth. These may come in a package in the store, such as a plastic bag, but they are whole and unadorned. They are different from processed grains, which use only a small portion of the grain (the starchy part, which is missing most of the vitamins, minerals, and fiber). Examples of processed grains include white flour, white rice, and grains packaged with flavorings, such as flavored sugary oatmeal or rice with added sauce and flavorings.

Also, there is an intelligence to the way other cultures cook their carbohydrates that gives the body an advantage in dealing with the carbs. Many cultures add other elements to their meals—not the preservatives and processed sugars and fats we tend to add, but things like spices and herbs that enhance digestion and help normalize the blood sugar response. The additions also make carbohydrate-rich foods tastier without creating an extreme dopamine spike and addiction response and help normalize blood sugar levels following a meal rich in carbohydrates.

Consider, for example, the ingredients in the Prime Curry Powder recipe you are already using. Its spices help normalize blood sugar and insulin responses. (Amla is even a treatment for diabetes.)[1] In India, amla is part of the diet, which helps negate some of the problems Americans experience when eating carbohydrates without the benefit of these spices. Turmeric is used in India as a traditional prevention for the development of dementia, and modern research demonstrates that it does have a measurable effect on behavioral and psychological dementia symptoms.[2] India has lower rates of Alzheimer's disease than in the United States.[3] Yet the Indian diet is predominantly a carbohydrate-based one. Because we couple it with these and other anti-inflammatory, blood-sugar-moderating, antioxidant-rich spices, digestive dysfunction doesn't result, and by extension, neither does the brain dysfunction. Also remember, the traditional Indian diet does not include highly processed foods that change the gut intelligence and alter the way the body responds to carbohydrates.

That doesn't mean you can just sprinkle curry powder on your doughnut and be fine, of course. I'm talking about the combination of making healthy carbohydrate choices like whole grains and starchy vegetables like sweet potatoes along with spices that help the body manage them. Eating this way will allow you to live in a world where you aren't constantly afraid of healthy carbs. But even healthy carbohydrates need a smart gut in order to be properly digested, and not everybody (especially those who are elderly) can stomach too many.

What About Bread . . . and Gluten?

People love bread. There is something comforting and ancient-feeling about it. I don't know who first said "Bread is the staff of life," but it does feel like a dietary staple to many people. We have it as toast, with sandwiches, before meals, during meals. Most of the bread you see in the supermarket, though, is definitely not a product of whole foods.

In fact, bread is confusing, Many so-called whole-wheat breads contain white flour as the first ingredient, and then just a little bit of whole grain. Even 100 percent whole-grain bread is processed: the wheat is milled into flour, the flour is mixed with other things like yeast and sugar (and often preservatives and other compounds that make it palatable and fluffy, like dough conditioners and extra gluten). I recently found some bread that was relatively unprocessed, containing only sprouted whole grains, yeast, water, and salt. The consistency was nothing like bread you are probably used to, though. If you can squish a piece of bread into a tiny ball in your hand, it is not a whole food. True whole-grain breads taste a lot more like European breads: hard, grainy, chewy, and definitely not fluffy. I find them tasty—more complex and interesting.

One of the reasons I think people are so attached to bread is that its refined flour and sugar give you a dopamine spike. When your dopamine is normalized through The Prime, you may find you prefer real whole-grain bread. The point is not to give up bread altogether. Instead, heal your digestion and then eat bread made with whole grains and without added sugars, chemicals, and preservatives and see whether you can tolerate it.

Yet there is another serious point to consider here. Of all the grain proteins out there that you have to choose from, there is one that I recommend being particularly cautious about. It also happens to be extremely pervasive in our food supply. It's gluten, and it is the protein in wheat, barley, and rye. It is not only in any food that contains these grains, but is often extracted and added to many kinds of food, such as soy sauce, salad dressing, and canned soup, not to mention every single white flour product on the shelves: cookies and crackers, bread and bagels. Many commercial breads include not just wheat but added gluten.

There are good reasons to back off from gluten or even avoid it entirely, especially as you are healing your gut on The Prime. Even with a smart gut, gluten is not completely digested—humans just don't have the enzymes necessary to digest the large amounts of gluten in the wheat available today. If your gut is not abnormally permeable and your detox pathways are not overloaded, most people can handle gluten in moderation (and by moderation I do not mean daily—*I mean weekly at most, and ideally no more than a few times a month*). Why is modern wheat so different? First, we consume way more than we should, so we are getting a much higher exposure than is normal. Wheat is in a huge number of processed foods, and many people are accustomed to eating a lot of bread, crackers, bagels, pasta, and baked goods.

Also, most of the wheat available today has been hybridized and has new properties so that it is no longer the same wheat that was discussed in ancient texts, and it contains significantly more gluten than in the past. Even if you are getting organic wheat products, there is often cross-contamination (from the wind and bees, which don't know the boundaries of an organic and nonorganic wheat farm), so it is really hard to say whether you are eating truly healthy wheat.

In Ayurveda and other ancient traditions, wheat flour was used almost immediately after grinding because it was known to quickly become rancid from the oxidation process—typically within two weeks. The wheat flour we use in our food is almost always much older than this. If you feel like you may be reacting to some food following The Prime and don't know what it is, try going gluten-free for at least one month and see if you feel better. If you do, it's time to take gluten off the menu, at least until your digestion is extremely strong. After that you may be able to eat gluten from a high-quality source every week or two—or you may react to it forever, in which case, it's not worth the price.

Tame Your Sweet Tooth

People love sugar, but they also tend to view it as "bad" or "sinful." What a conundrum—we shouldn't eat what we want the most? In Ayurveda, however, the view of sweets is a bit different. Sugars are considered medicinal in certain instances. "Sweet" is one of the six tastes in Ayurveda and plays an important role in digestion. In India, sugar is often in the form of jaggery, which comes in dark, crystallized chunks of unrefined cane sugar. It is often added to Ayurvedic formulas to help normalize neurological conditions; it has a strong flavor and you can't eat much of it. For this reason, foods that are sweet are not considered inherently "evil" in the way many people perceive white sugar, and they are not even contraindicated for someone trying to lose weight.

There is nothing wrong with sugar, in its natural form, and in small amounts. The problem (just as with wheat) is our culture's drastic refining and overconsumption of the stuff. The sugar most people eat today contains none of its naturally occurring nutrients.

Sugarcane juice naturally contains calcium, chromium, cobalt, copper, iron, magnesium, manganese, phosphorous, potassium, zinc, and vitamins A, C, B1, B2, B3, B5, and B12, plus many other naturally occurring compounds we haven't even named yet. What a waste that we throw all this away! When overconsumed, processed sugar is the most dangerous of all the carbohydrates in terms of the damage it can do to your gut and, by extension, your brain. But I say this not to demonize sugar, but instead to clarify so that you can make peace with your sugar consumption. You can learn to enjoy it in its natural form, in small amounts, once in a while, so that it becomes a treat not only for your taste buds but for your body as well.

You have already gone a long way in this direction with The Prime. Chances are, your sugar consumption has already been reduced spontaneously. You may want to go further. Now that you are curbing your cravings and regulating your blood sugar, you are ready to make some informed and lasting decisions about what sweets *you* choose to eat.

I suggest you make changes slowly for maximum effectiveness. Here are the steps I recommend. Do these one at a time and move on only when you feel comfortable with the step.

1. **Switch from refined and artificial sugars to natural sugars** most of the time. This is a pretty easy step if you eat most of your sugar at home, harder if you are still buying your sugar "on the outside," in the form of pastries at the coffee shop or candy from the vending machine. Try avoiding desserts unless you make them yourself using natural sugars or you have found a good source that uses natural sugars. You can even bring homemade sweets to work or on the road with you, to keep you away from candy bowls, vending machines, and the pastry case at the coffee bar. Examples of natural sugar include organic coconut palm sugar, unrefined cane sugar (such as jaggery and Sucanat), date sugar, honey, and real maple syrup. As you make this transition, you will likely find that your taste for sugar reduces. These natural sugars

are more satisfying because they also contain nutrients. I remember as a kid in India, we couldn't overeat sugar. The taste of the jaggery was too strong. A little was all we needed or wanted. Also remember that the less refined a sugar is, the less it will stimulate your addiction centers, so you won't feel compelled to eat more and more.

2. **Reduce your natural sugar intake.** A good goal is to enjoy a sweet treat with added sugar about once a week, but if you are having sugar every day, try cutting it out one day a week at first and moving forward from there at a pace that makes you comfortable.

3. **Reduce your grain intake.** Even whole grains have an impact on insulin and while I do not advise eliminating whole grains from your diet, cut back if you eat them at every meal or you eat large portions. Eating this way will also help your body to adjust and your blood sugar and insulin to rise and fall in more moderate waves. Also make sure to couple your grains with Prime Curry Powder as often as possible.

4. **Reduce or eliminate fruit juice.** Fruit is full of fiber and nutrients, but fruit juice is almost pure sugar, even if it is freshly squeezed and contains no added sugar. When the pulp and fiber are removed, the natural sugar in the juice quickly floods your bloodstream, which can have a similar effect to that of refined sugar, stimulating your addiction centers and making you want to eat more. If you love juicing, your juice should be 90 percent vegetable juice and 10 percent fruit, like the Prime Juice recipes. In my house, fruit juice is like candy to my son. Once a week, he gets to choose a sweet treat, and he often chooses fruit juice.

5. **Reduce your fruit servings to two to three per day.** Fruit is another excellent, nutritious food, but it does contain a lot of natural sugar. Enjoy it, especially for dessert as you are reducing your added sugar servings, but don't go too crazy with it if you are trying to lose weight. They say fruit is "nature's candy,"

and eventually you may find you don't want it all that often as your body adjusts and becomes more sensitive to sweet tastes. A fruit smoothie alone can have four or five servings of fruit, and that's a lot of fruit for one day. But if it's a choice between refined sugar and fruit, always go for the fruit.

Remember that these are general steps to work on when you want to do them and you feel ready. Don't let that punitive inner voice step in. If you have some chocolate, don't decide you have ruined it all. This is not about deprivation. This is about making changes you *want to make*, so proceed only when you feel ready. The amount a person needs to change his or her sugar consumption varies from individual to individual and depends on your Gut IQ after doing The Prime. These are only suggestions for those of you who feel like your gut could still use some extra support. Real and permanent change is a process, one that happens in a back-and-forth manner—two steps forward, one step back.

CLIMB THE SUGAR LADDER

If you want to improve the quality and minimize the toxicity of your sweetener choices, you can work your way up the ladder from the worst-quality sweeteners to the best. Job one: get off artificial sweeteners! Switch from artificial sweeteners to white sugar. Seriously. Even white sugar is better than the artificial stuff.

The one type of sweetener you should never, ever use is artificial sweetener. We know that artificial sweeteners are linked (counterintuitively) to weight gain[4] and to an increased risk of metabolic syndrome (prediabetes), higher than actual sugar provokes. One fascinating study linked this to the way artificial sweeteners alter gut microbiota, thereby inducing glucose intolerance.[5] I believe one of the ways this happens is that artificial sweeteners create inflammation, which alters gut flora and increases cravings, which result in eating more sugary comfort foods. Also, continuing to expose the palate to sweet tastes only encourages the desire for more sweet tastes.[6]

If you like stevia, you could switch to that next. It's an herb and I've never seen research stating it has any ill effects, but I'm personally not a fan. When using it, I detect an inflammatory effect in myself and with my family members. Skip that step on the ladder if you like, and move up to natural, unrefined sweeteners. Finally, reduce your intake of even natural unrefined sugar and, whenever possible, let fruit be your sweet treat. Take as much time as you need to, but keep climbing if you want to make a big impact on your gut bacteria as well as on your toxicity, inflammation, and energy levels.

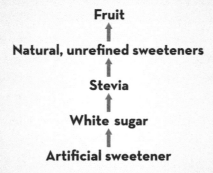

Fruit
↑
Natural, unrefined sweeteners
↑
Stevia
↑
White sugar
↑
Artificial sweetener

Note: Do not use honey in hot beverages or heat it by using it in baked recipes. When honey is exposed to heat, it releases a toxin called hydroxymethyl furfuraldehyde (HMF).[7] Heating also alters some of honey's other chemical contents, including increasing its peroxides. Finally, heating honey makes it harder to digest. The molecules become like glue, adhering to the mucous membranes and clogging all the channels in the body (called *srotas* in Ayurveda), which hinders detoxification and produces toxins (ama). Charak, the ancient sage of Ayurveda, once wrote: "Nothing is as troublesome as ama caused by improper intake of honey." For these reasons, I recommend keeping and eating your honey at room temperature or adding it to warm liquids/foods that are comfortable to touch.

Eat More Plant Foods

Plant foods such as vegetables, fruits, beans, nuts, and seeds can make up most of your diet, and as you progress in The Prime, you will probably want more of them as you may naturally desire less meat. Plant foods will make you feel good. They are highly nourishing and when they are organic, they are the least toxic foods you can eat.

Beans and other legumes (sometimes called pulses) such as lentils are excellent protein sources and a good example of how something can be partially processed but still whole-food-like and good for your gut. Beans that come in a can with only water and a little salt added are still close to their natural form. Dried beans are even closer, but they take much longer to prepare because they have to be soaked and then cooked. Rinse canned beans and enjoy them without much effort, knowing they are close to their natural state. Some people have trouble digesting beans, even if they love to eat them. In Ayurveda, beans and lentils are considered somewhat difficult to digest, but their overall health benefits still make them a good choice. The way that we counter this is to soak them for six to eight hours in water and add a pinch of fenugreek seeds while they are soaking. Then spices are added while they are cooking, such as Prime Curry Powder, to increase their digestibility. If you notice that you are having difficulty with beans and lentils, first try these hacks. If you are still having problems, then start with only split mung beans/lentils, and as your digestion gets stronger you can increase your bean and lentil intake. Many people find that as their digestive systems adjust to beans, they start making more of the natural enzymes that help digest them and beans are no longer a problem.

Choose Dairy Products Wisely

In Ayurvedic medicine, dairy plays a huge role in healing. In India, cows and cow products (milk, bovine colostrum, yogurt, ghee, and even urine) have special medicinal roles. Cows are revered in India because they are considered to be a manifestation of the healing Divine Feminine energy, and cow's milk is reportedly high in *ojas*, a liquid in the body recognized in Ayurveda as the source of health. You can think of ojas as the antidote for ama. A big part of what determines the presence of ojas in dairy products is the way that cows are treated—literally whether or not they are happy cows. So, in Ayurveda, when the healing properties of dairy products are discussed, it is with the assumption that they are coming from healthy, humanely treated cows that are living under natural circumstances.

Of course, in Ayurveda, they are also talking about the dairy available thousands of years ago, not the highly processed dairy products available to us today. Milk is treated much differently in India. For example, we would never drink cold milk. In India, as soon as you milk the cow, you boil the milk, turn off the heat, then serve it. The milk is creamy and sweet—as I mentioned in the first chapter, when we first moved to the United States, my sister and I couldn't drink the milk here for several years because it tasted so sour to us. I finally got used to it, but now I mainly drink raw milk typically in its fermented form: lassi.

Despite the fact that milk is less fresh in the Western world, it still has benefits. I advise choosing your milk wisely, however. Because my culture traditionally boils milk, I am not opposed to pasteurization, a process of heating the milk to kill bacteria. My recommendation is to buy raw milk, if you can get it, and boil only the small amount you plan to use, right before you are about to use it. Raw milk isn't processed the way other milks are, keeping it closest to its natural state as a whole food. It also has more of the natural enzymes and bacteria intact to help you break down the milk in your gut. Even my patients with severe milk allergies are often able

WHAT ABOUT FOOD INTOLERANCES
AND SENSITIVITIES?

Maybe you think you are intolerant to dairy or you are sugar-sensitive or gluten-sensitive or fat-sensitive or carb-sensitive. Maybe you are. And maybe you aren't.

Some people believe that feeling tired after eating or getting a stomachache is a sign of a food sensitivity—that they "can't eat carbs" or "can't digest fat." The strength of your digestion, however, determines the degree of your food sensitivities and intolerances. If you have really high agni, you can literally eat almost any food—this is the experience for most teenagers. As you get older, your agni goes down and you naturally get a little more sensitive to foods. Our culture has taken this to an extreme, however—and what we are seeing now in the United States is unprecedented. We have engaged in so many unhealthy habits that are killing our agni, and as a result our numbers of food sensitivities are exponentially higher. Add "new-to-nature" foods that our bodies don't recognize and it makes this problem even worse. Ignite the agni, fix the digestion, and many sensitivities you thought you had may resolve themselves.

This is where I feel that a lot of the health and diet books coming out that are targeting a single food group are really missing the point. In a weak digestive system, almost any food can become inflammatory and toxic. If you think you react to dairy or grains, maybe that's true, but you cannot know for sure until you heal your gut. If food particles such as milk protein molecules are leaking out into your bloodstream from your gut, your body will view these as foreign and you will have an immune response to them. But if those dairy molecules stay in your digestive tract like they are supposed to, you may not have any problem with them at all. I'm not saying I know that you won't, because some people will. Dairy *within* the digestive tract causes problems for some people (such as those with a lactase deficiency). But if you don't have a lactase deficiency, this may not be you. It may just feel like it right now, and it will continue to feel like it until you heal your gut. That's because some foods are toxic to you purely because of the way they aggravate what is already a problem.

It's a bit like salt on a wound. The problem isn't the salt. The problem is the wound. To really get to a point where your gut is healthy, you've got to heal this wound. Getting rid of the salt will help until the wound heals, but once healed, it won't hurt at all to rub salt on a healthy patch of skin. The Prime heals the wound and then allows you to decide based on your smarter gut's feedback what it can and cannot tolerate. Until your gut is healed, you will react to a lot of things. Once it is healed, you may find that only a few things cause a problem. In the case of dairy, especially when you are using healthy sources of dairy (organic, nonhomogenized, or raw dairy products) and only in moderation, you may find that the dairy you thought was a problem becomes a nourishing part of your diet.

to use raw milk once their gut is healed. There is a small risk of bacterial contamination with raw milk, but boiling takes care of this. In our home, we use raw milk occasionally, but I still boil it before I drink it, for digestibility. Mainly, I use raw milk to make homemade yogurt, which we use for lassi.

The bigger problem with the way we treat milk here is homogenization, which I find much more concerning. *Homogenization* is the process of breaking down the fat in milk into smaller particles so the cream doesn't float to the top and it looks the same from top to bottom. What is the point of this—to make the milk look prettier? The clumps of cream are the tastiest parts! The problem with homogenization is that once the fat is broken down into smaller particles, these particles can more easily escape the digestive system prematurely. They sneak under the digestive radar and enter the bloodstream undigested. I remember that when I switched from homogenized to nonhomogenized raw milk, I was able to digest it much better. If you think you have a problem with dairy, you may want to try this. It may just be that you need your dairy a little bit closer to its natural state.

From my own experience and by witnessing the experiences of thousands of patients who felt they had dairy intolerances, healing the gut and reintroducing dairy as raw milk often results in tolerance. With the reintroduction process, we go slowly. Often we never go back to the amount we were originally consuming, but smaller amounts work well for us. Another tip to help reintroduce milk into your diet is to boil it with a pinch of turmeric powder and a pinch of ginger (either powdered or freshly grated). This also makes milk more digestible (and tasty!).

Of all the dairy products I recommend, lassi is at the top of my list. Lassi is a diluted yogurt drink that is popular in India, and I highly recommend it for the probiotic assistance it offers your gut. Plus, it's delicious. There are two kinds of lassi: sweet and savory. Sweet lassis are flavored with natural sugars and spices such as cardamom powder and flavors such as rose water, but for the ultimate probiotic replenishment, I recommend savory lassi with digestive spices.

"SAY CHEESE..."

Can you guess the number one reason people cite for not being able to go vegan? It's cheese. You may love cheese, but you may not recognize how hard it is to digest, even under the best of circumstances. Cheese is similar to gluten in that it is never easy for anyone to digest and therefore should not be consumed in large quantities. Think about what cheese on a pizza looks like the next day: like a hard sheet of plastic, and it really won't change much even after days. It doesn't break down easily. If your Gut IQ is still a little low right now, cheese (and gluten) are best avoided, at least temporarily.

If you must have cheese, the best type is paneer, which is a homemade Indian cheese. It's really easy to make. Here's how:

Homemade Paneer

1/2 gallon raw, nonhomogenized organic milk
1/4 cup freshly squeezed lemon or lime juice

Heat the milk on the stove to about 176 degrees Fahrenheit (80 degrees Celsius), using a candy thermometer to get the right temperature.

Turn off the heat and stir in the citrus juice one spoonful at a time until curds start to form in the milk.

Let the curds cool for about 30 minutes; then strain and rinse them.

Paneer is often cooked with spinach or other vegetables in Indian cuisine, but you can also eat the curds plain if you are having a serious cheese craving.

As your gut heals and the bad bacteria die off while the good bacteria gain a foothold, you can help by introducing more good gut flora into the environment. You may wonder why I haven't had you taking probiotic supplements or drinking lassi earlier in the program. My patients often ask this, too, but the reason is that your gut wasn't ready. Until you clean up the gut and begin to reduce the population of bad bacteria, good bacteria you introduce won't be able to do anything. It would be a bit like sending Girl Scouts into World War II. The environment in your gut is just too hostile for their survival. Even yogurt is often still too hard on a healing gut, which is why I recommend lassi over straight yogurt. The added water and spices make the yogurt more digestible.

Ayurvedic medicine supports this point of view. Although certain fermented foods are helpful to a strong gut because of the good bacteria they contain, they can be difficult for an injured gut to digest. By discouraging the introduction of any fermented food (such as pickles of any kind, miso, tempeh, sauerkraut, soy sauce, vinegar, wine and beer, and even yogurt) while the gut is still healing, Ayurveda promotes a gentle environment in your gut. Once healing is under way, however, lassi is like dipping a toe back into healthy fermented foods. Because it is made with one part yogurt and three parts water (you can even make it more dilute than this when you first begin), it is easier on the gut and makes the yogurt more absorbable. If you have a dairy intolerance, I highly recommend making your own homemade yogurt using raw milk, starting with just 1 tablespoon of yogurt in a cup of water only once a week. Several affordable homemade yogurt makers are available even on Amazon if you want to try this (if you can't buy raw milk where you live, use nonhomogenized organic milk).

Another reason I like lassi is that the probiotics it contains are alive and thriving. When you take a probiotic capsule, how do you know how long it has been sitting on the shelf (three or four years?) or whether those bacteria are even still alive? With lassi, you know the bacteria are actively reproducing in the yogurt culture. Whatever your body gets in the form of a food, it will assimilate faster and more completely than what it gets in the form of a pill.

NONDAIRY LASSI

In general, lassi is best made with cow's milk because it contains the most healing properties. If you cannot tolerate cow's milk or dairy products, or your gut still needs a lot of healing, you can try goat-milk yogurt or coconut-milk yogurt to make your lassi. You can make your own yogurt using goat or coconut milk (you would need a starter or a little bit of yogurt, to get the bacteria going, just as you would when making cow's-milk yogurt). Or you can buy organic versions in the store, but avoid the sweetened varieties when making the digestive lassi.

There is a lot of research into probiotics, including research on the immune-stimulating[8] and weight-loss benefits of yogurt.[9] Now that you have tipped the scales in favor of the good bacteria in your gut, introducing lassi further supports the proliferation of a diverse and vibrant gut flora. You have created a home for the good bacteria to thrive, and now you are ready to reintroduce them to your gut.

I typically use two different lassi recipes with meals, but for gut healing, I recommend what I call digestive lassi. It isn't sweet and so will not trigger any healing or healed sugar addiction. Have this with lunch. It is too heavy to have later in the day. I make it about three times a week.

Digestive Lassi

Makes 1 serving

¾ cup room-temperature water
¼ cup nonhomogenized organic plain (unsweetened) yogurt*
½ teaspoon Prime Curry Powder, or to taste
(Optional: You can slightly roast the Prime Curry Powder in a
    skillet on the stove or in a toaster oven on aluminum foil and

> save it to use specifically with your digestive lassi, to give it
> an even deeper and more interesting flavor.)
>
> 1 pinch Himalayan salt

Put all the ingredients in a blender and blend until combined, or whisk with a fork. Enjoy with lunch.

*If your Gut IQ Test score was low, I would recommend starting with nonfat yogurt because it is easier to digest; start with a dilute version, using only 1 tablespoon yogurt in ¾ cup water. As you feel yourself getting stronger, you can switch to low-fat and eventually full-fat yogurt and slowly increase the amount of yogurt to ¼ cup.

The last dairy product I advocate is ghee. Ghee is clarified butter—it has all the milk solids taken out, so only the oil remains. Ghee is incredibly gentle, soothing, and calming, and it won't burn like butter so you can cook with it. A little ghee and Himalayan salt makes any grain or vegetable dish more interesting. I keep it in my kitchen cabinet all the time and use it anywhere I would use butter or vegetable oil. Ghee used to be hard to find in the United States, but it is now widely available in most well-stocked supermarkets.

There is one more aspect of dairy products that I would like to address. It may sound incidental to your health and weight loss, but it is actually relevant. I'm talking about the way the animal that provided the milk was treated. This discussion is relevant to the consumption of dairy, bone broth, and meat. Of course there is the ethical argument and animal cruelty, as well as environmental concerns, but there is a whole other factor, and that is the health of the animal. If the animals that provide milk or meat for your consumption are being injected with antibiotics and growth hormones throughout their lives, they are more likely to be sick animals. (Studies support the correlation of long-term antibiotic use and illnesses such as inflammatory bowel disease and cancer, as well as the idea that antibiotic use in food animals increases the development of antibiotic-resistant pathogens that put human and animal health at risk.) Many are concerned with growth hormone use as well. This is an area of ongoing research, and although one recent study suggested that bovine growth hormone has "little or no biological activity" in humans, a review of multiple studies found that it does have a harmful effect on the health of the cows. The use of bovine growth hormone (called rBGH) in cows increases their risk of mastitis, lameness, and reduced fertility. This isn't good for cows, but it's not good for people, either. This increase in mastitis (an infection of the udder) means that the milk produced by these cows contains increased antibiotics that are used to treat the mastitis.

The link between animal and human health isn't just about chemical residue, however. Remember that in Ayurveda, the mind and the body are linked. When animals are raised in stressful, cramped conditions, sometimes even literally being tortured, they have a physical response. Just as in humans, this stress causes a cascade of physical dysfunction that affects the body. Some of these feed animals, especially the larger ones, are quite intelligent and experience fear and stress (which don't require advanced intelligence). The conditions in which these animals are kept change the quality of the meat and milk because the biochemistry of the animal has changed in response to stress. When you choose a dairy or meat product, I recommend considering this seriously. Unhealthy, stressed animals are not a source for healthful food products.

In my family, we researched different dairies in California and buy dairy products from the ones that are the best in terms of animal welfare. A beginning step is to choose organic dairy products. A more advanced exploration would consider whether the animals are allowed to eat what they would naturally eat, whether they are pasture-raised or housed in enclosures, how often they get to move around, and how clean their environment is. I would rather limit animal product intake to those that have health benefits such as ghee and lassi, and be sure that what I do consume comes from healthy animals who don't require these disturbing interventions. This is also what I recommend for my patients, and you.

FLORA TONE

In addition to lassi, which helps repopulate your gut with friendly bacteria, I also really like and often prescribe an herbal supplement called Flora Tone from VPK (see Resources, page 293). Take it for eight to twelve weeks, starting with two tablets twice a day and working up to three tablets three times per day. This is a powerful way to further balance gut bacteria—so powerful that you may even notice a temporary return of detox symptoms as you have a large die-off of the bad gut bacteria. This will pass, and you will feel even better after it's over. I also recommend taking Flora Tone on an annual basis. Six to eight weeks per year is a good maintenance regimen.

I start some of my patients on a stronger program to help remove the parasitic bacterial overgrowth in their gut if they are still showing signs of imbalanced gut flora following The Prime. These programs are extremely individualized, however, because they often accompany quite significant bacterial die-off reaction and require close monitoring so that the liver doesn't get overwhelmed with the task of removing all the endotoxins released. I don't recommend those regimens in this book because you will need supervision, but Flora Tone is a great substitute for now. It is gentle and tolerated by most of my patients. If you feel you have bigger gut bacteria problems than you can handle on your own, I strongly recommend that you consult with an Ayurvedic, naturopathic, or functional medicine physician.

Reduce Meat and Fish Consumption (or Eliminate It)

Americans eat a lot of meat. Although meat eating works for some people and they feel they need it, others do just fine without it. I encourage a mostly vegetarian diet for many reasons, but one of the primary ones is that meat is hard to digest. The human body is not designed to process the large amounts of meat many people eat every day. Excessive meat consumption has many known health risks—expected ones, such as increased risk of death from heart attacks,[10] coronary artery disease, and stroke,[11] as well as surprising ones, such as increased risk of type 2 diabetes,[12] which is often thought to be more closely linked to excessive carbohydrate consumption.

Many studies have looked at the various typical components of vegetarian diets vs. omnivorous diets (containing animal products as well as plants) and found generally lower rates of cardiovascular disease, cancer (especially colon cancer), and obesity in vegans (who consume no animal products of any kind, including dairy products) and vegetarians.[13] One study looked at mortality in vegetarians vs. nonvegetarians and found significantly fewer deaths from ischemic heart disease in vegetarians. Vegetarians who included milk and eggs in their diets (lacto-ovo vegetarians) as well as those who also ate fish had death rates 34 percent lower than meat eaters. Death rates were 26 percent lower in vegans, and 20 percent lower in those who only occasionally ate meat.[14]

This may or may not convince you to cut down on meat, but chances are The Prime has already reduced your desire for large quantities of it. Most of my patients either spontaneously reduce their meat intake by about 50 percent on The Prime, or do so at this advanced stage upon my recommendation (when they want my advice on helping to identify which foods may be causing them to feel "toxic" from time to time). When they choose to reduce their meat consumption, they typically report that it is easy and in line with what they are feeling in their bodies. You certainly don't need meat in your diet, but if you want to continue eating it, you can do so.

The exception (as I have already discussed) is bone broth, which is much more digestible than meat and has a composition much more nutrient-rich than the muscle or flesh of an animal. I believe most people can benefit from the occasional use of bone broth, such as when they are going through a detoxification process, under stress, or just feeling physically exhausted. Even in India, when people are going through panchakarma (see Chapter 10) but are in a fragile state of health, doctors will have patients consume bone broth during the treatments.

The amount of meat products you can consume really depends on your body type and the state of your digestive system, but if you are going to eat meat, I strongly recommend choosing meat that is closest to its natural form. You want to avoid meat from a sick animal, from animals fed food that is not natural or native to them, and animals that are held in spaces not natural for their normal disposition. Anything else should not, in my opinion, even be an option. If the animal isn't healthy or is suffering, its meat will be toxic.

One obvious example of this is that stressed animals have muscles depleted of glycogen reserves. Glycogen is important to the industry because when levels are high in muscle tissue, lactic acid develops after slaughter, and lactic acid retards bacterial growth. Stressed animals deplete their glycogen reserves and therefore don't produce much lactic acid after slaughter, so they have meat that is much more likely to spoil while in storage and cause food poisoning.[15]

Many animal husbandry experts also believe that stress and suffering change the vitamin, mineral, and protein content of meat, as well as affecting texture, tenderness, color, and shelf life.[16] Just as in humans, an animal's state of stress and disease determines whether it is healthy or filled with endotoxins—just as we are filled with endotoxins from unhealthy bacteria in our gut when we are sick or stressed. These endotoxins aren't broken down through the cooking process. They are resilient. The meat industry is struggling with how to deal with this endotoxin issue. One idea was to create "maggot meat spray" and add it to the meat—so gross! When I refer to meat as a whole food, I'm really referring to meat that has not been highly processed and also to animals who have lived a healthy lifestyle. In my opinion, any meat that doesn't meet that definition isn't whole food.

Despite research on meat consumption, there is still a lively and ongoing debate about whether humans should eat meat and how much they should eat. Some research questions whether all meat should be studied together. Grass-fed meat from free-ranging or pastured animals and cured meat filled with preservatives and produced from factory-farmed or industrial feed-lot-confined animals are typically studied together, but some new research suggests that these types of meats have different effects in the body. Grass-fed meat contains much higher levels of omega-3 fatty acids, the brain-friendly type of fat that most Americans don't get enough of, as well as other beneficial fats such as conjugated linoleic acid and antioxidants. Grass-fed meat also contains more stearic acid, which doesn't raise cholesterol, while grain-fed and feed-lot meat contains more palmitic and myristic acids, which are the types of saturated fat more likely to raise cholesterol levels.[17] Bottom line: if you decide to continue eating meat, make sure your meat is coming from healthy animals.

Prime Food Swaps

To sum up, there are many simple ways you can swap out the foods you are eating for similar foods that have a much denser nutrient profile and are health-enhancing rather than health-destroying. Here are my favorite substitutes:

Instead of this:	Try this:
Butter or margarine	Grass-fed, organic ghee (clarified butter, or butter without the milk proteins). Many studies show benefits to cholesterol and other blood lipid factors with moderate amounts of ghee (between 5 and 10 percent of the diet).[18]
White table salt	Natural salts—such as sea salt and especially Himalayan salt. This pink-tinged salt is mineral-rich and free from the many industrial chemicals used to process white table salt. It comes from salt mines in the Himalayan mountains. In Ayurvedic medicine, we add this salt to the diet to treat inflammatory and autoimmune conditions.
White sugar and/or artificial sweetener	Coconut palm sugar, jaggery, turbinado sugar, or honey. Sugar is not supposed to be white!

As you consider this food guidance, please remember that it is always okay to go slowly. Don't get upset if you intend to reduce or eliminate something and then you have it anyway. This is all part of the process. Slow change is more permanent change. More than anything else, it is important to pay attention to your body's cues. You will continue to get better at this as your gut gets smarter and smarter. When you want something, try a little and see how you react. If something makes you feel tired or bloated or acidic or gives you a stomachache, notice that and remember it next time. If it helps you to remember, write it down. You can even turn your cravings journal into a food reaction journal where you track what you eat and how it makes you feel. This could be instructive, as you may determine patterns you didn't realize were there—foods your body loves and foods that don't agree with you. You are growing and changing and evolving as your body gets stronger and healthier. Let that happen and you will know exactly what you need to eat. Best of all, that's also what you will *want* to eat. The changes will be spontaneous.

CHAPTER 9

KNOW YOUR CONSTITUTION TYPE—AND EAT ACCORDINGLY

Now that you have some basic dietary principles to consider, the thought may have crossed your mind that perhaps not everyone does well eating in the same way. This is quite true. Maybe you have noticed that some people do quite well, for example, on a vegan diet, while others do not. Some thrive eating animal protein, while it doesn't work for others. There is a good reason for this. It all has to do with individual constitution.

You may remember (if you are of a certain age) when it was popular to categorize body types into ectomorphs, mesomorphs, and endomorphs. The ectomorph type tended to be narrow, thin, and tall. Mesomorphs were proportional with good muscle development, while endomorphs tended to be softer and rounder. The idea was that you couldn't fight your body type, but you could optimize it. Ayurveda has been using this concept for centuries, but in a more detailed and complex way. In Ayurveda, these types are called *doshas*, and three of them loosely correspond to the ectomorph, mesomorph, and endomorph types. Doshas, though, also take into consideration many other features, such as temperament and personality, habits and preferences, skin and hair color and texture, and much more. Body type is one important indicator of dosha, but it is only one part of the picture.

This ancient knowledge was obtained through close study of

human types, tendencies, and physical, mental, emotional, and spiritual traits, as well as the science of what helped and did not help them. There is no modern scientific equivalent to the doshas (the cutting-edge field of endobiogeny is looking at quantifying this ancient system), but I see the qualities lining up perfectly in my clinic all the time, and the food and health advice for each dosha always improves my patients' health profiles when they begin to follow it.

Your dosha (in other words, your constitution) provides a template for a much more individualized approach to self-care. The reason this is so important is that once you have cleared out your system and you are feeling better and stronger and healthier, knowing your dosha and what it means for your food and lifestyle choices can help you further tweak and hone your journey. Although for many people, simply clearing out ama and switching to whole foods will be enough, this is the chapter for you if you want to go even further, and especially if you have completed The Prime, made the changes suggested in Chapter 8 regarding whole foods, but still notice that you are having occasional toxic reactions to foods and still can't identify the source. You may be reacting to foods that are not suited to your dosha.

Diagnosing Your Dosha

The three doshas are called *vata* (similar to the ectomorph), *pitta* (similar to the mesomorph), and *kapha* (similar to the endomorph). Every human being is considered a mixture of these three types with their corresponding qualities, although typically, in any one person, one or two doshas tend to predominate. You may be pure vata, but more likely you are vata-pitta or vata-kapha. You may be all pitta, but you probably have a lot of vata or kapha qualities. Maybe you will learn that you are mostly kapha but have a nice helping of vata or pitta characteristics. (In a few rare cases, people are an even mixture of all three.) The subtle combinations and concentrations of these three types account for the myriad differences we see in each other—pretty cool, right?

Doshic tendencies manifest as physiological and emotional traits and trends in the body, and now that you are through all four stages of The Prime, you are likely detecting these more acutely than you did before. You are noticing what agrees with you and what doesn't, what you need to do and what doesn't feel right. These all relate to your unique combination of doshas.

I bring them up now because this is generally the point at which my patients want to go deeper. They want to explore their own tendencies and traits. They want to refine their diets even further. Your dosha can guide you. You may *feel* that (for example) you need or want hot soup and tea all day, but you may *think* you are supposed to be eating salads. If you discover that the vata dosha predominates in you, you will recognize that warm, comforting, rich foods are exactly what you need, and that cold raw foods will aggravate your constitution. Even the most pure and healthy whole-food diet will not work the same way in everyone. Your dosha determines the details.

DOSHAS AND SCIENCE

The notion that people have different physiological and psychological profiles poses a conundrum to scientists (or it should!), especially those, like me, who are also treating patients. Whenever some new health information comes to light, there is typically a fraction of the population that it works for, and a fraction that it doesn't seem to help at all, and a fraction that seem to get worse from it. When I am asked to interpret a study in terms of how it translates to what someone should do, my first question is: well, what type of people were being studied, and what is their Gut IQ? The individual differences in the people studied is the reason why you see, for example, some people thriving on a vegan diet while other people wither, and some thriving on a paleo diet while others can't stomach it. Certain antidepressant medications work for some people but not for others. Statin medications seem to help some and harm some. And when it comes to individual foods, the variations seem endless in terms of what agrees with whom. What is medicine for one can be poison for another.

One area of research that I think will eventually address this is epigenetics. Epigenetics is just now starting to come out with proof that environment affects gene expression. The doshas just add another layer. We are each a combination of genes, and our environments can turn those genes on or off. Our doshas, our constitutions, further influence how any given environmental aspect will impact any given gene. It's fascinating stuff and science is getting closer and closer to this understanding.

Ideally, eventually, modern medicine will realize that when you are conducting studies, you have to have a truly homogenous genetic population with similar digestive states and similar doshas in order to have reliable results. Even then, the results will be relevant only to the particular population you studied. Western medicine is in the early stages of understanding this.

So what is *your* dosha? This is the quiz I use in my seminars to help people determine their predominant dosha(s). You could get much more complex than this—some quizzes are much longer and go in more depth. I find that this one does a pretty good job of determining your general tendencies. The best way to determine your dosha is by seeing an Ayurvedic practitioner in person, but this can get you started. Once you know your type, I'll give you a description of the qualities of your dosha(s) and then I'll give you some specific dietary and lifestyle recommendations. Remember, these are just suggestions. These are tools you can use to continue on your journey. Go slow and incorporate the ones that feel right to you. I promise you will notice a difference once these customized foods and habits become a regular part of your life.

Dosha Quiz

FRAME
A. I am thin and slender with prominent joints and lean muscles.
B. I have a medium, symmetrical build with good muscle development.
C. I have a large or stocky build.

SKIN
A. My skin is dry and rough.
B. My skin is warm, reddish in color, and easily irritated.
C. My skin is moist and oily.

HAIR
A. My hair is dry, brittle, or frizzy.
B. My hair is fine, thin, or prematurely gray.
C. My hair is thick and wavy.

EYES
A. My eyes are small and active.
B. I have a penetrating gaze.
C. I have large pleasant eyes.

JOINTS
A. My joints are thin and prominent and have a tendency to crack.
B. My joints are loose and flexible.
C. My joints are large, well knit, and firm.

BODY TEMPERATURE
A. My hands and feet are usually cold and I prefer warm environments.
B. I am usually warm, regardless of the season, and prefer cooler environments.
C. I am adaptable to most temperatures but do not like cold, wet days.

STRESS
A. Under stress, I become anxious or worried.

B. Under stress, I become irritable, intense, or aggressive.

C. Under stress, I become withdrawn or depressed.

SLEEP
A. I am a light sleeper with a tendency to awaken easily.

B. I am a moderately sound sleeper, usually needing less than eight hours to feel rested, but I have vivid dreams.

C. My sleep is deep and long, and I tend to awaken slowly in the morning.

WEATHER
A. My least favorite is cold weather.

B. My least favorite is hot weather.

C. My least favorite is damp weather.

WEIGHT
A. I tend to lose weight easily.

B. I maintain my weight easily.

C. I gain weight easily.

APPETITE
A. On a daily basis, my appetite varies and I have delicate digestion.

B. I feel uncomfortable if I skip a meal and I can eat almost anything.

C. I like to eat, but can skip meals easily, and I have a slow digestion.

BOWEL MOVEMENTS
A. My bowel movements tend to be hard with occasional constipation.

B. My bowel movements tend to be loose with occasional diarrhea.

C. My bowel movements tend to be well formed or sticky with occasional constipation.

PERSONALITY
A. I am lively and enthusiastic by nature. I like change.

B. I am purposeful and intense. I like being efficient and in control.

C. I am easygoing and caring. I like to support others.

ACTIVITY

A. I like to be active and it can be hard to sit still.

B. I enjoy activity that has a purpose, especially competitive.

C. I like leisurely activities and staying home.

WALK

A. I walk quickly.

B. I have a determined walk.

C. I walk slow and steady at a leisurely pace.

MOODS

A. My moods change quickly, with a tendency toward anxiety.

B. My moods change slowly, but I can become angry easily.

C. My moods are mostly steady and most things don't bother me.

MEMORY

A. I learn quickly and forget quickly.

B. I have a good memory.

C. I learn slowly but have a good long-term memory.

ORGANIZATION

A. I am good at getting things started but not at getting things done.

B. I am organized and can focus on a project from start to finish.

C. I need help getting things started, but I am good at seeing things to the finish.

MONEY

A. I spend money almost as quickly as I make it.

B. It is important for me to have money and I spend it on expensive, luxury items.

C. I don't like to spend money and prefer saving it for a rainy day.

IN RELATIONSHIPS I USUALLY ASK . . .

A. What is wrong with me?

B. What is wrong with you?

C. Are you sure there is something wrong?

OUT OF BALANCE, I FEEL LIKE . . .

A. A leaf in the wind.

B. A raging inferno.

C. A bump on a log.

MY MOTTO IN LIFE IS . . .

A. Throw caution to the wind and live for today.

B. No pain, no gain.

C. Don't worry, be happy.

Count how many times you chose A, B, and C, and put the numbers here:

A: _____

B: _____

C: _____

If you have mostly A's: You are primarily vata.

If you have mostly B's: You are primarily pitta.

If you have mostly C's: You are primarily kapha.

If you have a pretty close score in two areas, then you are likely a mix of those two types, with your higher score being the slightly stronger dosha. If you have an almost exact three-way split, you are what is called tridoshic, a balance between all three types (this is unusual but possible). After the following descriptions of the doshas, I will explain how to manage the sometimes conflicting recommendations when you have high or nearly equal numbers for two doshas or all three doshas. Let's begin by talking about what it means to be each type.

Vata

In the slide presentations I give, I choose some characters that represent classic versions of each dosha. The classic vata type is Audrey Hepburn or, if you prefer cartoon characters, the Road Runner. Vatas tend to be slight, wiry, and fine-boned, but there are exceptions, especially when vata is out of balance and develops low agni (i.e., a dumb gut). In this case, they can develop subcutaneous, squishy, loose fat. This is not natural for this type of body frame.

When balanced, vatas are quick to catch on to things and highly creative and intuitive. Out of balance, they can be anxious and nervous and may experience insomnia and constipation. Excess vata can mimic or even eventually lead to neurological issues, including dementia in old age, because the area where vata imbalances become most concentrated is in the colon—the digestive organ that houses the most gut bacteria and therefore exerts the strongest impact on the nervous system.

Vatas tend to be irregular in every way when they are out of balance. They have irregular digestion, irregular sleep patterns, and irregular moods. This is the mood-swing dosha! Vatas can be hungry, then completely forget to eat. They may sleep too much or not be able to fall asleep at all. They tend to have worse PMS symptoms than other doshas. (Around the time of the menstrual cycle, most women have a temporary increase in vata energy.) This is why vatas benefit more than any other dosha from a calm and regular routine. Warm, rich foods and calm situations balance vata.

Too much exercise is overstimulating, and most vatas don't need much. They are already full of energy. Restorative yoga poses that focus predominantly on stretching are particularly good for vata. Calm regularity is the order of the day.

When a vata gains weight, it tends to be the squishy, soft, subcutaneous kind of fat that pulls away from the muscle. This kind of fat also tends to be quite visible on small-framed vatas, and it makes them self-conscious. Vatas also tend to be the most vocal about their weight gain. Aesthetically, vatas hate extra fat because they have naturally thin bodies so it feels out of balance, but in the early stages, it's really the least harmful type of fat accumulation because it is all on the surface.

Ironically, in the early stages, the same processes that make vatas lose weight become what make vatas gain weight. For example, coffee and cold water are touted for their weight-loss benefits and may have this effect temporarily in vatas, but eventually they will cause such vata aggravation that they can have the reverse effect because they will significantly and negatively impact digestion to the point that the person begins to accumulate ama.

To calm and pacify vata, focus on:

- Warm, cooked foods
- Hot beverages
- Soft moist foods such as pasta, cooked cereal, and soup
- Oily foods, such as those containing ghee (clarified butter), oil, nuts, or avocado
- Sweet foods

Foods Good for Vata

GRAINS
Oatmeal
Quinoa
Rice (basmati rice and brown rice)
Wheat (nonmodified)

LEGUMES
Red lentils
Tofu
Whole mung bean soup
Yellow split mung beans

VEGETABLES
Artichoke
Asparagus
Beet
Carrot
Mustard greens
Pumpkin
Spinach
Sweet potato
Yams
Yellow squash

DAIRY
Butter
Buttermilk
Cheese (soft, non-aged only, such as ricotta, cottage cheese, and paneer)
Ghee
Lassi
Milk (served warm)

SWEETENERS
Cane sugar, whole natural form only (such as Sucanat)
Date sugar
Honey
Jaggery
Maple syrup
Molasses

OILS
All

NUTS AND SEEDS
All nuts, except peanuts
Seeds in small amounts

SPICES
Anise
Bay leaves
Black pepper
Cardamom
Cinnamon
Clove
Cumin
Fennel
Fenugreek
Ginger
Himalayan salt
Lemon juice
Mustard seeds
Tamarind

FRUIT
All sweet, juicy fruits
Apples and dried fruits are best
    cooked or stewed
Apricots
Bananas
Berries
Cherries
Figs
Grapefruit
Grapes
Lemon juice
Lemons
Limes
Mangoes
Melons
Oranges
Papaya
Peaches
Pears
Pineapple
Plums
Pomegranate
Note: Dried fruits should be
    soaked prior to eating

MEAT
Eggs
Fish and seafood
Poultry
Red meat

To avoid aggravating vata, stay away from:

- Light, dry, crunchy foods

- Cold foods

- A completely vegan lifestyle. Vata is the only dosha that sometimes requires some animal protein when it gets out of balance, but most vatas tend not to want much. If a vata really can't do meat, consider at least including organic raw nonhomogenized dairy and free-range eggs from humanely raised sources and chicken bone broth.

Foods to Avoid for Vata

GRAINS
Barley
Buckwheat
Corn
Granola
Millet
Raw oats (such as when it is
    added to granola)
Rye

LEGUMES
All except yellow mung beans,
    red lentils, and tofu

VEGETABLES
Alfalfa sprouts
Broccoli
Brussels sprouts
Cabbage
Cauliflower
Potatoes
Raw lettuce and salad greens
    (although vatas tend to love
    salads)
Raw vegetables of all types

SPICES
Any very hot spices, such as
    cayenne pepper and chili
    peppers
Raw garlic
Raw onion

FRUIT
Apples (if raw)
Cranberries
Dried fruits (if not soaked)
Unripe fruits

Vata Sample Meal Plan

Breakfast	Stewed apples with cinnamon, cardamom, and raisins
Lunch	Basmati rice with curried vegetables (such as asparagus and zucchini) cooked in ghee; roasted chicken
Snack	Dates, nut butter, fresh fruit (except raw apples)
Dinner	Lentil soup

Lifestyle Hacks to Keep Vata Balanced

- **Keep regular hours.** Get up and go to bed at the same time on most days, and have your meals at the same time on most days. Regular habits are difficult for vata to maintain, but they are calming and balancing.

- **Get enough sleep.** Vatas need the most sleep of all the doshas, about nine hours per night.

- **Stay warm and moist.** Cool, dry conditions are aggravating to vata. Wrap up in blankets and drink warm tea in the winter. On warm sunny days, however, go out and bask! Vatas love the sun.

- **Practice gentle moderate exercise,** such as walking and yoga. Vatas like gentle calming yoga and may also really enjoy hot yoga.

- **Manage anxiety and notice nervous habits.** Meditation and deep breathing are pacifying for excess vata energy.

Pitta

Pittas are high achievers, ambitious and driven. Martha Stewart is a good example of a pitta, and Yosemite Sam is a good example of an out-of-balance pitta. Too much pitta energy can cause anger, irritability, and a red face. When pittas gain weight, it tends to be inflammatory weight, with lymphatic accumulation and Fake Fat. On The Prime, pittas in particular drop weight quickly as lymph begins to move more quickly and inflammation cools.

Pittas tend to run hot, both literally and metaphorically. Physically, they are average, with medium build and good muscle development. They tend to have blond or red hair, early balding or thinning hair in women, piercing eyes, and sharp voices. They can be intimidating. They are good at winning arguments.

Pittas benefit more than any other dosha from time in nature. Nature is incredibly rejuvenating and calming to pittas, the perfect remedy for irritation and anger. Pittas also need to stay cool, to balance their hot temperaments. Cool weather is made for pittas. They are often warm in the winter when everyone else is freezing. They should aim for moderate exercise but can get too competitive in sports.

When pittas gain weight, I call it "angry weight." A lot of pitta weight is related to inflammation—it comes with pain, discomfort, joint aches, and rashes. It's not squishy weight like vata weight. It is inflammatory weight, consisting of a lot of water retention that holds the excess heat so characteristic of pittas. It is the most uncomfortable kind of weight.

Pittas are particularly prone to lymphatic backup, or Fake Fat. All the heat and inflammation collect in that water and lymph. This is why pittas do so well with cooling foods that turn down the heat and allow that water to start coming out. On The Prime, you have already done a lot to help reduce inflammation, so the process has begun. For pittas, it is especially important to limit key foods that increase heat.

Because pittas tend to be healthy and have the strongest digestion of all the doshas, they are most likely to be able to get away with eating toxic foods when they are younger. However, once the inflammation starts and their gut becomes permeable, it all goes downhill until the digestion is healed again and the inflammation is cooled. Alkaline foods will most enhance this effect. Pitta is the one dosha that can do well with raw foods once digestion is healed, especially in the summer at lunchtime. Hot weather is a challenge with pittas, but cooling raw foods will reduce inflammation in a healthy pitta gut.

If they can just keep the heat down and the lymphatics moving, pittas can become extraordinarily productive people. They are creative and goal oriented and they have a lot of energy.

To calm and pacify pitta, focus on:

- Juicy foods, such as grapes, mangoes, lettuces, and cucumbers
- Cooling foods, such as kale, arugula, melons, and coconuts
- Foods with high water content
- Room-temperature to lukewarm drinks

Foods Good for Pitta

GRAINS
Amaranth
Barley
Kamut
Oats
Quinoa
Rice—white, specifically
    basmati, jasmine, Texmati

Wheat (nonmodified and in moderation, such as less than weekly)

LEGUMES

Chickpeas

Kidney beans

Mung beans

Nonfermented soybean products (tofu and edamame, not tempeh—fermentation makes the food more heating to the body, which pittas should avoid)

Split peas

All other legumes are okay in moderation, such as red beans and orange, yellow, and black lentils

VEGETABLES

Alfalfa sprouts

Artichoke

Asparagus

Bok choy

Broccoli

Brussels sprouts

Cabbage

Cauliflower

Celery

Chard

Cilantro

Cucumber

Green beans

Green leafy vegetables (all except spinach)

Kale

Lettuce

Okra

Parsley

Peas

Potato

Sweet potato

Winter squash

Yellow squash

Zucchini

DAIRY

Butter

Cream

Cream cheese (in moderation)

Ghee

Lassi, sweet (as opposed to savory lassi, mentioned in the last chapter, sweet lassi is spiced to make it sweet and more pitta balancing)

Milk (served heated on the stove—you can allow it to cool to lukewarm if you prefer)

Paneer

SWEETENERS

Cane sugar, whole natural form only (like Sucanat—but in moderation)

Coconut palm sugar

Date sugar

Jaggery

OILS

Coconut oil

Ghee

Olive oil (in moderation)

Sunflower oil (in moderation)

NUTS AND SEEDS

Almonds (blanched only, in small amounts)

Coconut

Pumpkin seeds (in moderation)

Sunflower seeds

SPICES
Cardamom
Cilantro
Coriander
Cumin
Dill
Fennel
Mint
Rosemary
Saffron
Turmeric

FRUIT
Apples
Dates
Figs
Grapes
Mangoes
Melons
Oranges, sweet
Pears
Persimmon
Plums, sweet
Pomegranate
Raisins

MEAT
Chicken (white meat only)
Egg whites
Fish (freshwater types only, such as trout, catfish, walleye, and tilapia)
Turkey

To avoid aggravating pitta, stay away from:

- Spicy foods

- Sour foods

- Acidic foods, such as vinegar

- Salty tastes

Foods to Avoid for Pitta

GRAINS
Brown rice (short grain)
Buckwheat
Corn
Millet
Rye

VEGETABLES
Beets
Carrots
Onions
Radishes
Seaweed
Spinach
Tomatoes and their products (such as tomato sauce, salsa, and ketchup)
Turnips

DAIRY
Cheese (especially aged and salty, such as feta and blue cheese)
Sour cream
Yogurt

SWEETENERS
Honey
Molasses
Processed white sugar

OILS
Canola
Corn
Mustard
Peanut
Safflower
Sesame

SPICES
Asafetida (also called hing, a
  common spice in India)
Bay leaves
Black pepper
Cayenne pepper
Chili peppers
Fenugreek
Garlic
Ginger
Horseradish

Ketchup
Mustard
Mustard seeds
Paprika
Soy sauce

FRUIT
Berries
Cherries
Grapefruit
Lemons
Limes
Olives
Peaches
Prunes
Sour fruits of any kind

MEAT
Beef
Egg yolk
Lamb
Pork
Seafood

Pitta Sample Meal Plan

Breakfast	Oats with raisins, shredded coconut, and a little coconut palm sugar
Lunch	Soup, rice, beans and lentils, vegetables, leafy greens (except spinach), animal protein (if not vegetarian), even dessert like rice pudding. Pittas like a big lunch—it keeps them calm for the rest of the day.
Snack	Melons, coconut water, dried coconut
Dinner	Roasted vegetables and grains

Lifestyle Hacks to Keep Pitta Balanced

- **Stay passionate and creative.** Pittas need something to be ambitious about, but they can take ambition too far. Instead, focus on passions, which channels pitta energy in a more productive way. This will help you work better with others and focus competitiveness into a common goal.

- **Get enough sleep.** Pittas need about eight hours per night to stay friendly and not be irritable and snappy.

- **Practice short bursts of fast-moving exercise,** such as running, hiking, swimming, or biking. Pittas are good sprinters. Outdoor activities are especially enjoyable and balancing for pittas. But because of their competitive natures, pittas can sometimes overexert themselves.

- **Practice awareness about what you say and how you say it.** Pittas can be sharp-tongued and hurt other people's feelings unintentionally. Noticing this and modifying your response is therapeutic for pittas (and can improve relationships). It's great to be ambitious and smart, but not so great for your personal life or your career goals to be a perfectionist and intolerant of others.

- **Avoid being a workaholic** and make sure you make time to play.

Kapha

Kapha is the relaxed, mellow, chill dosha, and people who are predominantly kapha have a let-it-be approach to life that naturally isn't prone to stress, anxiety, irritation, or any of the emotions that tend to put people off. This is why kapha types are usually so popular—everybody likes the person who doesn't sweat the small stuff. Oprah Winfrey is a good example of a kapha type. She has a calming, positive presence that makes people feel good. A cartoon example is Winnie the Pooh—a cheerful, happy, likable bear who is perhaps overly fond of honey.

Physically, kaphas tend to have the most difficulty keeping weight off. They are usually big-boned and sturdy and they can go for long periods without eating. However, they truly enjoy their food, and sugar and dairy in particular are weaknesses that only make their weight accumulation worse. This is the only dosha that does well with any sort of fasting on a regular basis.

They also tend to be congested and have sinus issues. They have great endurance (should they choose to use it) and make good long-distance runners. They tend to have smooth, luminous skin, glossy dark hair, lovely singing voices, and good memories. When out of balance, they can lack motivation, feel too lazy to do anything, and lie around a lot, snacking on sweets and cheese.

A sedentary lifestyle is particularly attractive to kaphas and they really have to gear themselves up to get off the couch and move around. Kaphas benefit from moving and eating light, stimulating foods to combat the tendency toward malaise and overindulgence. Vigorous exercise is good for them. They benefit most from warm, dry climates, such as desert environments, to combat their naturally cool and wet constitutions.

When kaphas gain weight, it is aesthetically pleasing weight. Because kaphas are naturally big-boned and structured, weight gain adds a reassuring substance. However, this is also the most dangerous kind of fat because it deposits around organs, such as in the heart. In the beginning, kaphas can gain weight and you don't really see it. It doesn't stick out and look obvious like vata weight. Kaphas will seem as if they just keep expanding—getting bigger and even more beautiful, staying smooth and voluptuous. This has historically been viewed as beautiful weight, like in the old paintings. However, this weight is the hardest to lose and the most likely to contribute to the slow development of chronic disease. Because it is dangerous weight, kaphas should work on reducing it so the organs don't begin to carry the extra load.

The problem with kaphas and fat isn't a question of modern aesthetics and the fat shaming that goes with it. Instead, it is a matter of health. Even balanced kaphas tend to have fat deposits in the organs. For this reason, kaphas have to be especially rigorous about monitoring their weight. If you think you are a kapha, you should weigh yourself every week, because you may not even notice any change in your body but the scale can reveal when your weight is climbing. For the sake of your health, you must be vigilant. This is one of the reasons why a low-fat vegan diet is so crucial for kapha health. Low-carb diets recommending high fat are disastrous for them. Kaphas even have to be careful with grain consumption because grains are heavy and sweet (in Ayurvedic terminology) and increase kapha.

Kaphas need a low-fat, vegan, nutrient-rich, low-calorie diet with limited fruit. It's the hardest to follow, but a kapha will thrive on it. When kaphas break their addiction cycle to food, they are the naturally healthiest people on the planet. They have strong immunity, they are balanced and calm, and if a meteor hit the earth and all the food was gone, the kaphas would be the ones to continue the human race.

To calm and pacify kapha, focus on:

- Warm cooked foods
- Dry foods, such as popcorn and rice cakes
- Light foods, low in fat and oil
- Hot or warm beverages
- A vegetarian or especially vegan diet

Foods Good for Kapha

GRAINS
Aged grains (allowed to age
   for at least one year before
   processing and eating,
   making them more digestible)
Barley
Buckwheat
Corn
Millet
Oats
Quinoa
Rice
Rye

LEGUMES
All legumes, such as lentils,
   kidney beans, split peas,
   chickpeas, and adzuki beans.
   Generally avoid tofu unless

it is a choice between tofu and meat, in which case tofu is the superior choice for kaphas.

VEGETABLES
Artichoke
Asparagus
Beets (small amounts)
Broccoli
Cabbage
Carrots
Cauliflower
Celery
Eggplant
Green beans
Green leafy vegetables
Okra (only dry-fried; don't cook until not slimy)
Onion
Peas
Peppers
Potatoes
Radishes
Sprouts
Zucchini

DAIRY
Buttermilk
Ghee (small amounts)
Lassi (savory, not sweet)
Low-fat or nonfat milk (in moderation—a couple of times a week at most)

SWEETENERS
Honey

OILS (ALL IN SMALL AMOUNTS)
Canola
Corn
Flax seed
Mustard
Safflower
Sunflower

NUTS AND SEEDS
Pumpkin seeds
Sunflower seeds

SPICES
All spices, except salt

FRUIT

Note: Of all the doshas, kapha people, as well as anyone with a kapha imbalance (as indicated by carrying excess weight), must be the most careful about fruit. Sweet tastes aggravate kapha, and especially kaphas who are trying to lose weight. They should limit fruits to just one or two servings per day.

Apples
Apricots
Cranberries

Dried fruits
Pears
Pomegranates

To avoid aggravating kapha, stay away from:

- Large quantities of food, especially at night
- Heavy food

- Cold food
- Watery food
- Sweet, sour, and salty tastes
- Cold beverages

Foods to Avoid for Kapha

GRAINS
Grains that are not aged
Oats
Rice
Wheat

LEGUMES
Tofu (but this is still preferable to meat for kapha)

VEGETABLES
Avocadoes
Sweet potatoes
Tapioca
Yams

DAIRY
Butter
Cheese
Cream
Ghee in large quantities
Ice cream
Sour cream
Whole milk
Yogurt

SWEETENERS
All sugarcane products

OILS
All oils in amounts larger than 1 teaspoon per day

NUTS AND SEEDS
All nuts

SPICES
Salt

FRUIT
Bananas
Coconut
Mangoes
Melons
Oranges
Pineapple
Plums

MEAT
Kaphas should avoid all meat, because of their slow digestion and tendency to gain weight.

Kapha Sample Meal Plan

Breakfast	If you aren't hungry, skip breakfast, or have some herbal tea. If you are hungry, try dried fruit, stewed apples, or millet porridge.
Lunch	Dry-sauté vegetables with curry mix and little oil. Add onions, garlic, peppers, black pepper, and just a touch of Himalayan salt—not much! Add any grains and/or legumes you like from the preceding list of kapha-approved foods.
Snack	Kaphas do best if they avoid snacking, but if you really need a snack, have some pumpkin seeds or unsalted popcorn.
Dinner	Kaphas typically don't need dinner, but an early bowl of vegetable or lentil soup can stave off hunger if it arises. For most kaphas, digestion is at 0 percent after 7 p.m., so eating late is especially hard on them.

Lifestyle Hacks to Keep Kapha Balanced

- **Get moving!** Kaphas need to stay stimulated or they may not do much of anything, because sitting and relaxing is so enjoyable to them.

- **Don't oversleep.** Kaphas need the least sleep of all the doshas in order to feel good, but they tend to sleep more than is needed. Kaphas typically need only seven hours or even less per night, so they can and should wake up before 6 a.m.

- **Get deep tissue massages.** These are great for kaphas, whose systems need stimulation because everything tends to run slowly, including digestion and the lymphatic system.

- **Let it go.** Although kaphas are the mellow, let-it-be types, they can also be possessive and overly thrifty when out of balance. They hold on to things and don't ever want to let go or allow change. They can tend toward hoarding. Practicing awareness about nonattachment is good for kaphas. Remember that everything is temporary and life moves forward like a river, rather than sitting like a stagnant pond.

This is a good thing, although sometimes hard for kaphas to accept.

What If You Have Two or Three Predominant Doshas?

Most people have more than one predominant dosha. If you are a vata-pitta, vata-kapha, or pitta-kapha, how do you know which dosha to balance, which foods to eat, which qualities to nurture? First of all, be sure you read the sections on both of the doshas that are dominant in you. You will need the information from both.

Next, work on balancing the dosha that is most out of balance at the moment. You probably know which one it is. You can tell this by which dosha-relevant qualities are most aggravating you. For example, a pitta-vata person should focus on pitta when feeling hot, irritated, or overly harsh with people, but on days when that same person feels more anxious, nervous, jittery, or ungrounded (such as during travel or PMS), vata-balancing should be the focus. A vata-kapha person, to use another example, may focus on vata-balancing during travel or when feeling anxious but should switch to kapha-balancing when feeling dormant, lazy, or unmotivated, or in the case of weight gain. A kapha-pitta, to use another example, may usually focus on kapha foods to keep weight down and energy up, but sometimes, when irritability takes over, or when feeling heated, pitta balancing should prevail. Remember, we all have all three doshas in us, and even the least dominant dosha can sometimes flare up and cause a problem. It's good to know how to balance them all.

When all doshas feel pretty balanced, it's best to focus on those that are most dominant according to the season. During the summer, focus more on pitta; during fall and early winter, focus more on vata; during late winter and spring, focus more on kapha.

TRENDY DIETS AND DOSHAS

There are a lot of diets out there, and the reason why they work so well for some people and not others has everything to do with the doshas. For example, I have patients in my clinic who do the paleo diet and feel great, while others try it and don't feel well at all. Someone who is predominantly pitta may eat a lot of berries, spinach, acidic foods, and red meats on the paleo diet and get aggravated, whereas the animal protein in the paleo diet may be calming and grounding to a vata type. You can generally modify most special diets you like (vegan, alkaline, paleo, or whatever it is) for your type, based on the food lists and other principles I've provided, but in general I find that certain types of diets go best with certain doshas:

- **Vata:** This is the only type I believe does well on a **paleo diet** long-term, and the only type that can benefit from small amounts of animal protein on a regular basis. Vatas need to be grounded. They need more weight, and animal protein keeps them there, while all the vegetables and fruits on the paleo diet can be tailored to vata's particular needs. Ironically, the worst diet for vata is the raw diet, which is highly aggravating, and yet many vatas feel compelled to eat salad all the time.

- **Pitta:** Because pitta runs hot and also acidic, pittas do well on an **alkaline diet**, which emphasizes mild, cooling, alkaline foods such as leafy greens, cucumbers, celery, peas, apples, and melons. Of course, pittas tend to crave meat and highly spicy food, which is quite aggravating for them if eaten regularly. Pittas should moderate their intake of meat because it is so heating to the body, and they should be particularly cautious about gluten because these are both inflammatory for a pitta's already overheated gut. Once digestion is healed, pitta is the dosha that does best on occasional raw foods, such as having a salad for lunch.

- **Kapha:** Kapha is the one dosha that truly thrives on a **vegan diet**. The light, stimulating foods are just the ticket for getting kapha up off the couch to spread her cheerful demeanor and wise counsel far and wide. Of course, kapha is the dosha least likely to *want* to eat a vegan diet. They crave meat and dairy, but they really are natural-born vegans and if they eat a vegan diet, it is unbelievable how good they will feel. Kaphas on vegan diets can live to a ripe old age because kaphas are so naturally sturdy. Kapha is the only dosha that really never needs any animal products, other than bone broth during periods of cleansing and healing. Light grains and cooked veggies are the ultimate kapha diet.

Do You Really Need to Balance Your Doshas?

After The Prime, if you are eating whole foods and continuing with your progress, you are noticing your body more, your habits are changing spontaneously, and you feel pretty good, you may not feel the need to change your diet to be dosha-specific. This is totally fine. Eating for your dosha at this point is only for those who feel like they are still having problems and want more help. How strictly you need to follow these dosha guidelines really depends on your Gut IQ. Once your gut heals, you can "violate" these dosha rules and still feel fine most of the time because your agni can assimilate a diverse whole-food diet.

What I notice, though, is that over time (typically a course of three to five years), if maintenance continues and people continue to redo The Prime annually as a cleanse, their bodies tend to get pulled naturally in the direction of these dosha-specific foods. There is also a natural tendency to prefer the seasonal foods. In other words, if eating for your dosha feels too strenuous or like too much of a stretch right now, don't worry about it. It is certainly not a requirement. Just bookmark this chapter, and take another look at it once every year or so. You will probably notice, eventually, that you are moving toward these recommendations spontaneously, at least seasonally.

There is no rush. Don't force any of these changes. Only follow them when you feel compelled to do so. This chapter is provided solely as a reference to you, for when you start wondering what may be going on as your gut continues to get smarter and smarter. These recommendations are a reflection of how your gut wants to eat in accordance with your specific constitution. But you have to be ready for them. When you are, these foods will feel and taste right to you and it won't take any effort to choose them.

CHAPTER 10

MORE AYURVEDIC WISDOM FOR THE REST OF YOUR LIFE

You've come a long way. You've made great progress. You've accomplished many things, but at this point, you may be inspired to go even further. You could add hundreds of practices, habits, and interventions to your lifestyle and routine that will continue to facilitate and maximize your health and your body's ability to capture nutrients and detoxify effectively. Getting your digestion working is really only the beginning of the journey. Where you go from here is entirely up to you.

Maybe you are fine with the routine you've set up for yourself; great! I find that many of my patients want more information at this point. They have questions about things they have heard of and they want to know if these practices will help them. For this reason, I have created this chapter to share the health practices I endorse. These are the icing on the cake, the things you may want to try adding every so often, like when you are making a New Year's resolution or feeling the urge to do some physical spring cleaning.

You may not have heard of some of the things in this chapter. They are mostly ancient techniques that have been modernized for use in the twenty-first century, but they are Ayurvedic in origin. They also work. If I'm not sure something is effective, or if I don't have experience with it, it's not in this chapter. These are things you can do to continue to increase your healing and become even more energetic, sharp-minded, and healthy. You probably won't try all the techniques in this chapter, but I hope you'll at least read about them and try out a few to see how they may fit.

Try Oil Pulling and Tongue Scraping

Oil pulling has become trendy lately in holistic health circles, but it is certainly nothing new. It is an ancient Ayurvedic practice designed to clean bacteria out of the mouth and between the teeth—bacteria that could otherwise be easily released into the bloodstream. Many studies show that oral bacteria can enter the bloodstream through several mechanisms and cause or contribute to serious health problems, most notably cardiovascular disease.[1] Studies have also noted a correlation between poor oral hygiene and cardiovascular disease.[2] Oil pulling is a natural, nonchemical way to reduce these bacteria.[3]

Oil pulling does more. It is a routine method of daily detoxification. The underlying theory behind oil pulling is that there is a two-way exchange in the mouth: substances can go in and they can also come out, as they do through the skin. This is why we give some medicines and vitamins sublingually: it is an effective way to absorb substances into your bloodstream immediately. Ayurveda takes this one step further, recognizing that the tongue and all the tissues of the mouth can also excrete substances from the body; the mouth can pull stuff out through the salivary glands, helping to cleanse both the lymphatic system and the blood. Sesame oil, in particular, can increase this detoxifying effect, but coconut oil is a good oil to use, too.

You may have heard a lot of bizarre claims that oil pulling can cure all kinds of health issues, including depression and acne. Let me be frank and tell you that there is no clinical evidence for this. There is a lot of anecdotal evidence, however, that has accumulated over thousands of years. This is not sufficient to convince some people that oil pulling is worthwhile, and I understand that. I also know that people tend to exaggerate or misunderstand the effects of treatments like this. Keep in mind that when you are doing an Ayurvedic treatment such as oil pulling, you are never doing just that one thing. You are doing a combination of things that have a cumulative effect on the body. If your acne clears up or your depression lifts, it's not just the oil pulling, but it could be the cumulative effect of many interventions that include oil pulling. The dental hygiene effects are straightforward, but the systemic effects are interwoven with everything else you are doing.

Still, I believe that oil pulling does what Ayurvedic medicine says it does: it provides a gentle, simple detoxification of the tissues of the mouth and of the entire body, which can and does excrete toxins through the mouth. Any gentle detoxification that you do may be extremely mild in its effect if you do it once, but it can become powerful if you do it on a daily basis over time.

After oil pulling, the oil you spit out should be white and foamy. That means you are doing it correctly. Don't just hold it in your mouth. Swish it around! Keep it moving. After you spit it out, you may notice a thick coating on your tongue. This is another sign that you are doing it correctly. At this point, after you rinse out your mouth, you may want to clean your tongue with a tongue scraper. (I'll explain how shortly.)

You don't have to practice oil pulling and tongue scraping every day, but regularity is key for any Ayurvedic practice. (I do this when I'm at home and my schedule is normal, as part of my regular routine.) At first, it may feel bizarre to you—the oil is a strange texture in the mouth if you aren't used to it. If you don't like it, try doing it three times a week. If you can do it every day, that's even better, but three times a week will still make a difference. You don't have to devote any real time or attention to it. Just do it. I typically do it while I'm in the shower. I come out, spit, scrape, and brush my teeth. You don't have to sit there and just swish it around, wasting time. Do other things and then spit it out.

If you have dental hygiene problems such as halitosis (bad breath), gingivitis (inflamed gum tissue), or receding gums, I would strongly encourage you to oil pull every day. I have treated patients facing thousands of dollars' worth of dental work just with oil pulling. Once my patients feel like their gum health has normalized, they tend to want to keep it up because they never want to go back to that place. Also, the oil pulling gives you an even cleaner feeling in your mouth than just brushing and once you get used to that, your mouth feels dirty when you don't do it.

Oil Pulling Instructions

Oil pulling is easy. All you need is 1 to 2 tablespoons of sesame oil. You can also use sunflower oil or gently warmed coconut oil (to make the coconut oil liquid, if you prefer that—otherwise it will liquefy in your mouth) if you don't tolerate sesame oil. For most people, sesame oil works best.

Swish the oil around in your mouth, sucking it through your teeth, for up to twenty minutes. Do not swallow any of the oil, which is pulling toxins out of your body. You may need to start with just one or two minutes, until you get used to doing it and are able to hold the oil in your mouth for longer periods of time. After you are done, spit it out and scrape your tongue, then brush your teeth.

Tongue Scraping

You could brush your tongue with your toothbrush, but research shoes that a tongue scraper is much more effective, reducing volatile sulfur compounds on the tongue by 75 percent, compared to just 45 percent with a toothbrush.[4] Most people have a light tongue coating, but take a look at the tongue of a small child (or someone with strong digestion). There will be a little coating toward the back, but the tongue is very red or pink. As we age and have more built-up ama, this is reflected on the tongue.

All it takes to scrape your tongue is a tongue scraper and a few minutes. You can buy a tongue scraper at most pharmacies and discount stores, as well as at health food stores and online. Stick out your tongue and place the scraper as far back as you can. Using gentle pressure, scrape down to the tip of your tongue. Rinse the scraper and repeat until the tongue looks clear of coating. Do this on most days, after oil pulling and before brushing your teeth. Most people are shocked by the amount of residue that comes off their tongue in the beginning, but as you clean your tongue on a more regular basis, it will have less of a coating over time.

Go Microwave-Free

This one may sound really radical to you, but here it is: Dump your microwave oven. Really! It may sound like an impossibility—how would you warm up your tea, reheat your leftovers, make day-old pizza edible again?—but hear me out. There are some good reasons why microwaving may be hurting your health. I haven't owned a microwave for ten years and I would never bring one back into my house. Here's why:

- If you have a microwave, you are more likely to eat processed food, which is filled with "new-to-nature" chemicals such as preservatives and colorings and highly processed food. If you eat frozen, microwaveable food, getting rid of your microwave will make you more likely to get into the kitchen and cook the real stuff. That alone is reason enough, in my opinion, to stop the microwave madness.

- Microwaving fosters the idea that food should be convenient and you should prepare and eat it as fast as possible. If you can make a meal in two minutes and eat it in three minutes, your digestion is going to have a hard time keeping up. Humans digest food much better when they spend time washing, chopping, cooking, looking, smelling, tasting, seasoning, serving, sitting down, and savoring their food. This gives your body a chance to fully prepare to receive food (prereleasing all the right enzymes in response to smell and taste), and you will be more likely to chew more thoroughly, pay closer attention to what you are eating, and enjoy the whole experience more. This will be more fulfilling, and for that reason, you may end up eating less,[5] or at least not over-eating and overtaxing your digestion.

- Finally, let's discuss the most controversial position: that microwaving alters the molecular composition of food in a way that renders it less nutritious and even toxic. The scientific literature hasn't fully figured this one out yet, but there is evidence that microwaving does change food in ways that regular cooking doesn't. For example, one study showed that microwaving protein solutions caused the proteins to unfold at a much higher rate than with ambient heating.[6] Other studies show mixed results for things like vitamin, mineral, antioxidant, and other phytochemical substances, especially in vegetables. What are we to make of all this? The answer is that modern science doesn't yet have an answer, so their answer is that microwaving is safe.

Ayurveda has a different answer. Most people agree that microwaved food *tastes different* from food cooked on a stove or in the oven. It changes the texture of, for example, pizza crust or the bun in that leftover half sandwich you brought back from the restaurant. Rice gets dry. Pasta gets gummy. Vegetables can shrivel into a weird shadow of their former selves. Of course, one could say that this happens when people don't use the microwave correctly. But many people don't know how to use the microwave to best advantage, and what's happening to the food they eat from that magic box in the meantime? In Ayurvedic medicine, food is alive, but when we alter it at the molecular level, it becomes "new to nature," and our bodies don't necessarily understand how to process it. This can hinder digestion, and anything that hinders digestion is to be avoided, Ayurvedically speaking. For that reason, I consider the microwave off limits. Even if science hasn't proven it yet. But maybe you want more proof.

Try cooking a potato in the microwave, and another one in the oven. Taste them together and see if you can tell the difference. Another visual I give my patients is: put a piece of bread in the toaster and then put another in the microwave. The toasted bread is crispy and tasty. The microwaved bread is like rubber, and when it cools, it becomes hard as a rock. Let your kitchen be a laboratory. If you don't have the scientific proof, make your own.

And what better proof than what your own body can offer you? Try going one month without eating anything from the microwave; then reintroduce it and notice how you feel. At this point, you have developed the body awareness to notice how microwaved food affects you. Your sense of taste is sharper and you are more aware of how you feel after eating foods. I bet you can tell the difference. Eat something from the microwave and pay attention to what your body says.

To this day, if I eat something microwaved (which typically happens at someone else's house—we sit down, they are committed to organics, the food looks great), I get terrible stomach bloating and something doesn't feel right. The scientist in me has to know, so I sometimes ask, "Did you happen to microwave any of this food?" Sure enough, the answer is always yes.

There are many arguments in favor of microwaves, and I have heard them all. It's faster! (Really? It doesn't take much longer to heat water on the stove or in an electric kettle than in a microwave. It is just as quick to heat pizza in the toaster oven as in a microwave.) It's more convenient. It's cleaner. It takes fewer dishes. None of these are worth the potential health sacrifice, in my opinion. Microwaving has become a cultural habit, but once you get used to not using it, you won't miss it.

Experiment with Enemas

Called *bastis* in Ayurvedic medicine, enemas are considered an ancient and important part of purification therapies like panchakarma (which I'll tell you about a little bit later in this chapter). Bastis are so important because of the important role of the colon in processing end-stage toxins. Sometimes, things get stopped up in there, and bastis can be helpful in getting them moving out of the body.

Although I've talked about the digestive system as a tube, it certainly isn't a straight shot from beginning to end. It twists, it turns, and it folds back on itself over and over. Microscopically, even the folds have folds. These folds are useful for peristalsis—they allow the muscles to move them, accordion-like, so they can push food through. However, the downside to this structure is that food and old stool and bacteria can get trapped in all those folds. There are some really obvious manifestations of this—conditions such as toxic mega colon, in which someone is so constipated and waste builds up to such an extent that the colon stretches almost beyond its limit and the bacterial load becomes life-threatening. However, on a more subtle level, slow movement and buildup can be more than uncomfortable. It can be toxic in a more low-grade, chronic way, as the bad bacteria aren't shed quickly enough and accumulate in the colon.

An enema will clean out the lower colon. A colonic—which always should be administered by a professional—cleans higher up, which means it can be more detoxifying but also harsher. In some circles, these have become quite popular as health maintenance practices, but an Ayurvedic enema has a specific method behind it: First, the enema cleanses and nourishes with a substance such as chlorophyll or other herbs, and then it is always followed (the next day or in the evening of the same day) by an oil enema, to relubricate the colon and help dissolve some of the lipophilic (fat-loving) toxins that won't dissolve in water. You would never do a water enema without getting an oil enema afterward because water alone strips away moisture and good bacteria. The bowel is moist and needs to stay lubricated with fats and mucus to hold the good bacteria. It's not supposed to be squeaky clean.

I recommend doing an enema about twice a month (good for those who are having a really hard time detoxifying), and never during the menstrual cycle for women. Once a month is plenty for people who are not having trouble detoxifying. There are special purification protocols in Ayurveda when enemas are done more frequently, but those are always under supervised conditions.

But perhaps you are squeamish about this practice. Perhaps you are thinking, "No way would I ever do that!" I felt the same way when this was first prescribed to me by my Ayurvedic physician. When I started traveling more and experiencing more discomfort in my body, I decided I should try it. I couldn't believe how good it felt to do this once a month. I felt like it really invigorated my entire system, including my lymphatic system. It relieved premenstrual discomfort, lowered my inflammation, and even improved my mood. (Enemas stimulate the vagus nerve, which as you now know is linked to the brain. They also get rid of a lot of the bacteria that can make you feel poorly.) And for anyone who has skin conditions, the chlorophyll enema is a godsend. I recommend that people with skin conditions add chlorophyll enemas twice a month either during or following The Prime until the skin condition resolves.

If monthly is still too much for you, I suggest at least trying this twice a year, for a spring and fall cleanse. A lot of my patients who would never in a thousand years have thought they would be doing enemas, especially male patients, later tell me they hate to admit it but they feel fantastic afterward. The first time is usually the least comfortable because there is an initial detoxification reaction. You may feel crummy for a few days, but don't let that discourage you. It only gets better and better, and if you feel bad at first, it is evidence that the intervention was particularly needed.

Here are instructions for how to do a chlorophyll enema, and how to follow it with an oil enema.

How to Do a Chlorophyll Enema

Supplies:

- Disposable enema bags (available on Amazon)
- Organic Liquid Chlorophyll by World Organic (also available on Amazon)

Preparation of the Chlorophyll Enema:

- Warm 3 cups of filtered water (see the following directions for details).
- Add 3 tablespoons of liquid chlorophyll to the warm water.
- Empty one to two capsules of probiotics into the mixture and stir (this step is optional but beneficial; choose any probiotic with at least 1 billion colonies—I prefer the ones in the refrigerated section of the store, as I believe these bacteria are more likely to be intact).

General Instructions:

- The water should be heated up to where it is slightly warmer than room temperature and still comfortable to touch. If you have overheated the water, just wait for it to cool.
- When you pour the mixture into the enema bag, the lock on the enema tube should be on.
- Lie on your right side and insert the enema tube 3 to 4 inches into the rectum. If the tube isn't prelubricated, you can use some coconut or sesame oil to lubricate it.
- Unlock the tube to allow the enema to move into the rectum.
- Lock the tube again once the enema has been administered and before you remove the tube from the rectum—this prevents leakage from the tube.
- Try to hold the enema for 5 to 10 minutes. Sometimes you have to administer a small amount (about 1 cup) and then

empty the bowels. Then administer the remaining amount and hold for 5 to 10 minutes. If it becomes uncomfortable at all, just empty your bowels. You can work up to 5 to 10 minutes. I don't recommend holding it any longer.

For the Follow-Up Oil Enema

- The evening of or the day after doing a chlorophyll enema, heat 1 to 2 cups of cured, organic sesame oil warmed to slightly warmer than room temperature. If you want to customize your oil enema for your dosha, use sesame oil for vata and kapha, but add 1 cup of coconut oil to 1 cup of sesame oil for pitta.
- To cure the sesame oil, add one drop of water to the oil and heat until the drop "pops." Once the oil cools, you can store it for future use.
- Administer the enema as above. You may need to wear a pad that day because occasionally there is some leakage of the oil during the day or night.

Note: Again, never do an enema the week of your menstrual cycle.

Fast Intermittently—but Only When It's Right for You

Fasting is trendy, especially something more recently being called intermittent fasting. Fasting is a general term for going without food for a set amount of time (from a few hours to a few weeks), with or without liquid additions. Sometimes fasting is used to refer to going without a particular thing, such as sugar, meat, or alcohol, but that's not the technical definition. Intermittent fasting is a more periodic type of fasting. While Ayurveda recommends that everyone should go for twelve hours without eating between dinner and breakfast for good health, intermittent fasting goes beyond this. There are many ways to do it, such as going for sixteen hours without eating. For example, if you finish dinner at 6 p.m., you would not eat breakfast until 10 a.m. For others, intermittent fasting means fasting for one day every week, or one weekend per month, or one week per year. The idea is that fasting gives the body a rest from digestion so it can concentrate on healing. This works for some people, in certain situations. For others, it is almost always a bad idea.

So how do you know whether fasting is right for you? First of all, I want to make one thing clear: Fasting, and intermittent fasting in particular, is an advanced technique. Most people don't need to do it, especially if they are practicing the aspects of The Prime and eating whole foods according to their unique constitution or dosha. If you don't ever want to fast, then don't.

Some have come a long way in their detoxification journey, however, and want to fine-tune their bodies and minds further. You must have your detoxification pathways turned on before fasting and you should be nutritionally replenished, or calorie restriction will not have a detoxifying effect. It will only have a depleting effect. If you are already efficiently detoxing and you want to try fasting, it could be valuable for you. I want you to understand, though, that fasting is more of a mental than a physical feat. Emotions come up strongly during a fast, which surprises many people. It helps to be prepared for that.

But should you fast, even if you want to? Before you make that decision, you must consider your predominant dosha:

Vata: Fasting is *not* appropriate for vata people most of the time. If you really want to do a fast, do it only in the spring, as the weather is getting warmer. During this time, I recommend fasting no more than one day a week for no more than four weeks. During that one-day fast, have Prime Broth or other warm soupy liquids for all three meals. You should never go without any food. Another option some vatas like is to skip just one meal, such as dinner, or eat only Prime Broth or soup for dinner. This can also be a gentle way to get the benefits of fasting without overly aggravating vata energy.

Anything more extreme will increase vata energy too much. You could feel highly aggravated, anxious, nervous, or hyperactive, and you can stop absorbing nutrients altogether and become nutrient-deficient quickly. Even if you enjoy this kind of heightened state, it is stressful on your body and mind. Calming is more important. A daily meditation practice is a much more valuable use of your time.

Pitta: Pittas can fast, but they don't generally like to because they have such large appetites. However, for pittas who overeat, occasional fasting can help keep things under control. The only caution for pittas is that fasting can increase the digestive fire (*agni*) a little too much. If you start to feel heated, aggravated, and irritable, it may be time to end the fast. Pittas need to fast only about once a month for regular maintenance and should *never* do a water-only fast. The best way for pittas to fast is up to one day per week for as long as they like. However, if this is long-term (more than four weeks in a row), they should only skip breakfast and dinner and should have something for lunch. Alternatively, a pure liquid diet of vegetable juice in the morning and Prime Broth for lunch and dinner would be appropriate one day per week for pittas. Pittas always need something in the middle of the day, even if it is only Prime Broth.

Kapha: This is the dosha that is built for fasting. Kaphas can comfortably go for extended periods without food, and it is good for their physiology to do this. When offered only healthy choices, kaphas naturally tend to eat little anyway. It's their cravings that get them into trouble. They are also the least aggravated, mentally, by fasting. Kaphas don't usually want to hear that they are good at fasting because they tend to be the most emotionally attached to food. However, fasting is easy for them, once their addiction pathways are normalized (i.e., after The Prime).

Fasting benefits kaphas in particular because it increases the number of mitochondria (the energy producers in cells) that are produced in the body, and fasting also increases the expression of the cytochrome P450 enzymes so crucial for detoxification. Because kaphas retain toxins and fat more stubbornly than other doshas and tend to have low energy when imbalanced, they particularly benefit from these effects. When kaphas fast, their whole system becomes more efficient. They can easily fast for a full twenty-four hours one day per week either on just water alone or on a full liquid diet. They can do it easily—but just remember that first they must normalize their food addictions and release their strong emotional attachment to food.

How hard would it be to skip one day of eating, or one meal, once a week or every so often? You may really enjoy the effects. Just be sure you are efficiently digesting first and you are in a nutrient-dense state. Keep up with your good habits. And never forget this, if you are even considering fasting—I cannot overstate the importance:

Fasting is *not* for when you've been practicing unhealthy habits and want to get back on track. It is *only* useful for when you are already on track and detoxing well. This is when fasting has a positive rather than a negative effect.

Also remember that intermittent fasting has health benefits, but severe calorie reduction on a persistent basis can be destructive to the body, especially if you have more of the vata and pitta physiology. Food is healing. It's good to eat!

Indulge in Panchakarma

I believe panchakarma should be on everyone's bucket list and covered by every medical insurance company. Panchakarma is a seasonal purification therapy involving a visit to a panchakarma center, where patients receive varying degrees of consultation, Ayurvedic diagnosis and prescription, and treatment, including yoga and breathing exercises, dietary recommendations and herbal prescriptions, traditional Ayurvedic massage (*abhyanga*), a treatment in which warm oil is poured onto your forehead (called *shirod-*

hara; this is extremely calming and relaxing), oil application to the nasal passages (*nasya*), herbal enema (*basti*), and often other treatments as well.

Normally, panchakarma treatments last anywhere from three to twenty-one days or even longer, depending on the severity of a particular health condition. I have sent some of my patients with chronic neurological conditions such as amyotrophic lateral sclerosis (ALS), multiple sclerosis, and Parkinson's disease to panchakarma with astounding results. I have been doing panchakarma every year for over a decade, sometimes even traveling to India for really deep treatments, and it has radically altered the way I have aged. I highly recommend it. It's also pleasurable—like a spa experience.

Panchakarma can do many good things for you. It relaxes you, it makes your skin glow, and it has even been shown to improve measures of both health and well-being. For example, people undergoing panchakarma demonstrated an improved ability to make behavior changes three months after the therapy.[7] There has also been research showing an improvement in cardiovascular risk factors after panchakarma.[8] I particularly like panchakarma because it can go even further than The Prime in digging deep down into those fat-soluble toxins and releasing them more effectively than any other intervention I know. In one study, researchers looked at people receiving five days of panchakarma. They tested blood levels of highly toxic PCBs (polychlorinated biphenyls, manufactured chemicals with documented health consequences including cancer) and Beta-HCH (beta-hexachlorocyclohexane, a by-product of insecticide production) before and after the therapy. The body can typically clear these toxins by a small fraction of 1 percent in five days. These fat-soluble toxins are the most difficult to remove and among the most dangerous in the body. With panchakarma, the toxins were reduced by 46 to 48 percent within just a few days.[9] No other detoxification method has been scientifically verified to reduce this amount of fat-soluble toxins in the human body in such a short period without causing negative side effects. Normally, these toxic compounds remain in the body for a lifetime. Panchakarma gets them out in an extremely short period of time.

Of course, it's not in everyone's budget or temperament to travel to India for a health treatment. Fortunately, there are an increasing number of good panchakarma programs in the United States, of varying lengths. I hope you will look into this treatment and consider it. For many of my patients, it has made a profound difference, and it is powerful for treating extremely difficult conditions. Panchakarma is one of the most nourishing, loving, and profound ways that someone can heal and detoxify.

If you are interested in doing panchakarma in India, my only caution is to watch out for "tourist panchakarma." Most of the truly authentic panchakarma places in India, where you get real results, are not in luxury hotels. Tourist-oriented places tend to offer the more superficial treatments, which are certainly enjoyable and relieve stress but won't get the deep level of detoxification that you can get in more authentic places. These authentic places can truly be life altering, and as a nice bonus, many people conclude panchakarma ten to twenty pounds lighter.

Staying Primed

At last we have come to the end of The Prime. You may have completed the program, but I hope you will not leave The Prime behind. In fact, you can live Primed all the time, and I hope you will. This is what I want for you: to achieve everything you are capable of achieving. You don't have to stick with every single habit you've learned every day of your life, but if you live your life doing the interventions that you really enjoy or that you feel make a difference for you at least five days per week, you will continue to make progress.

Detoxification is a lifelong and constant process, but health can be a state you live in from now until the end of your ripe old age. Stay mindful of your body. Pay attention to how you live and how it affects you. What happens in your body and mind when you eat different things, do different things, even think different things? You've done the work, but self-awareness lasts a lifetime, and self-nurturing should never end.

Most of all, remember that health has many sides and angles, each capable of glinting like every facet of a diamond, and health allows you to live your life fully awake and engaged. Life too is infinitely complex, and Ayurveda is the science of life. Let your own life be your source of study, your passion, and your ultimate motivation. The Prime is about being ready to live, but it doesn't end there. After you Prime yourself for health, the really exciting part starts: living your healthy life and finding out how far you can go, how much you can do, and how fully you can be who you really are.

This is living. This is the science of your life. This can be your great passion: how to live best. Once you have established that mind-body connection through The Prime, which helps you determine what is and what is not good for you, you can live this dynamic and ever-changing process with awareness and intelligence. You can become your own best expert. No one else understands your body as well as you do. You just have to wake up to its needs and break free of the biochemical chains that were dictating your actions before. You are on the right track because now you are Primed.

NOTES

Chapter 1: You're Doing It Backward

1. Agriculture Fact Book, Chapter 2, "Profiling Food Consumption in America": http://www.usda.gov/factbook/chapter2.pdf.
2. Yang Q, Zhang Z, Flanders WD, Merritt R, Hu FB. Added sugar intake and cardiovascular diseases mortality among US adults. *JAMA Intern Med.* 2014;174(4):516–24.
3. Malik VS, Schulze MB, Hu FB. Intake of sugar-sweetened beverages and weight gain: a systematic review. *Am J Clin Nutr.* 2006 Aug;84(2):274–88.
4. Johnson RJ, Segal MS, Sautin Y, et al. Potential role of sugar (fructose) in the epidemic of hypertension, obesity, and the metabolic syndrome, diabetes, kidney disease, and cardiovascular disease. *Am J Clin Nutr.* 2007 Oct;86(4):899–906.
5. Pereira MA, Kartashov Al, Ebbeling CB, et al. Fast-food habits, weight gain, and insulin resistance (the CARDIA study): 15-year prospective analysis. *Lancet.* 2005;366(9464):1030.

Chapter 2: Not Your Everyday Detox

1. Creamer B, Shorter RG, Bamforth J. The turnover and shedding of epithelia cells, Part I: The turnover in the gastro-intestinal tract. *Gut.* 1961:2,110.
2. "Background on Chemicals and Waste," United Nations Environment Programme: http://www.unep.org/chemicalsandwaste/ Introduction/BackgroundonChemicalsandWaste/tabid/1059847/ Default.aspx.
3. "Body Burden: The Pollution in Newborns," The Environmental

Working Group, July 14, 2005: http://www.ewg.org/research/body-burden-pollution-newborns.

4. Cohen J. Faster environmental testing for new synthetic chemicals and materials. *UC Santa Barbara Current*, Science+Technology section, April 10, 2014: http://www.news.ucsb.edu/2014/014070/faster-environmental-testing-new-synthetic-chemicals-and-materials.

5. Worldometers, which tracks toxic chemical release by industry on a real-time counter: http://www.worldometers.info/view/toxchem/.

6. Moreira MA, Andre LC, Cardeal ZL. Analysis of plasticizer migration to meat roasted in plastic bags by SPME-GC/MS. *Food Chem.* 2015;178:195–200.

7. Lim JS, Lee DH, Park JY, Jin SH, Jacobs DR Jr. A strong interaction between serum gamma-glutamyltransferase and obesity on the risk of prevalent type 2 diabetes: results from the Third National Health and Nutrition Examination Survey. *Clin Chem.* 2007;53(6):1092–109.

8. Brown RJ, DeBanate MA, Rother KI. Artificial sweeteners: a systematic review of metabolic effects in youth. *Int J Pediatr Obes.* 2010;5(4):305–12.

9. Suez J, Korem T, Zeevi D, et al. Artificial sweeteners induce glucose intolerance by altering the gut microbiota. *Nature: International Weekly Journal of Science.* 2014;514:181–6.

Chapter 3: Neuroadaptation, Food Addiction, and Your Brain

1. Barry D, Clarke M, Petry N. Obesity and its relationship to addictions: is overeating a form of addictive behavior? *Am J Addict.* 2009:18(6):439–51.

Chapter 4: It's Not What You Eat, It's What You Digest

1. "The Sensitive Gut," a Harvard Medical School Special Health Report prepared in consultation with Lawrence S. Friedman, M.D., 2012.

2. Alcock J, Maley, CC, Atktipis CA. Is eating behavior manipulated by the gastrointestinal microbiota? Evolutionary pressures and potential mechanisms. *Bioessays.* 2014 Oct;36(10):940–9.

3. Dutta G, Zhang P, Liu B. The lipopolysaccharide Parkinson's disease animal model: mechanistic studies and drug recovery. *Fundam Clin Pharmacol.* 2008 Oct;22(5):453–64.

4. WebMD article discussing the medical status of leaky gut syndrome: http://www.webmd.com/digestive-disorders/features/leaky-gut-syndrome.

5. Fasano A. Zonulin and its regulation of intestinal barrier function: the biological door to inflammation, autoimmunity, and cancer. *Physiol Rev.* 2011 Jan;91(1):151–75.

6. Fasano A, Shea-Donohue T. Mechanisms of disease: the role of intestinal barrier function in the pathogenesis of gastrointestinal autoimmune diseases. *Nat Clin Pract Gastroenterol Hepatol.* 2005:2,416–22.

7. Ch'ng CL, Jones MK, Kingham JGC. Celiac disease and autoimmune thyroid disease. *Clin Med Res.* 2007;5(3):184–92.

8. Visser J, Rozing J, Sapone A, Lammers K, Fasano A. Tight junctions, intestinal permeability, and autoimmunity celiac disease and type 1 diabetes paradigms. *Ann N Y Acad Sci.* 2009;1165:195–205.

9. Autoimmune statistics from the American Autoimmune Related Diseases Association, Inc.: http://www.aarda.org/autoimmune-information/autoimmune-statistics/.

10. Cyrex Laboratories, http://www.cyrexlabs.com.

Chapter 5: Leaky Brain: Understanding the Brain-Gut Connection

1. Camilleri M. Serotonin in the gastrointestinal tract. *Curr Opin Endocrinol Diabetes Obes.* 2009;16(1):53–9.

2. Corcoran C, Thomas P, O'Keane V. Vagus nerve stimulation in chronic treatment-resistant depression. *Brit J Psychiat.* 2006;189:282–3.

3. Alcock J, Maley CC, Aktipis CA. Is eating behavior manipulated by the gastrointestinal microbiota? Evolutionary pressures and potential mechanisms. *Bioessays.* 2014;36(10):940–9.

4. Collins SM, Surette M, Bercik P. The interplay between the intestinal microbiota and the brain. *Nat Rev Microbiol.* 2012 Nov;10(11):735–42.

5. Braak H, Rub U, Gai WP, Del Tredici K. Idiopathic Parkinson's disease: possible routes by which vulnerable neuronal types may be subject to neuroinvasion by an unknown pathogen. *J Neural Transm.* 2003;110(5):517–36.

6. Del Tredici K, Rub U, De Vos R, Bohl J, Braak H. Where does Parkinson's disease pathology begin in the brain? *J Neuropath Exp Neur.* 2002 May:61(5):413–26.

7. Holmqvist S, Chutna O, Bousset L, et al. Direct evidence of Parkinson pathology spread from the gastrointestinal tract to the brain in rats. *Acta Neuropathol.* 2014;128(6):805–20.

8. Van Oudenhove L, McKie S, Lassman D, et al. Fatty acid-induced gut-brain signaling attenuates neural and behavioral effects of sad emotion in humans. *J Clin Invest.* 2011;121(8):3094–9.

9. Prat A, Biernacki K, Wosik K, Antel JP. Glial influence on the human blood-brain barrier. *Glia.* 2001;36(2):145–55.

10. Ruhl A. Glial cells in the gut. *Neurogastroent Motil.* 2005;17(6):777–90.

11. Savidge TC, Newman P, Pothoulakis C, et al. Enteric glia regulate

intestinal barrier function and inflammation via release of S-nitroso-glutathione. *Gastroenterology.* 2007 Apr;132(4):1344–58.

12. Louveau A, Smirnov I, Keyes TJ, Eccles JD, Rouhani SJ, Peske JD, Derecki NC, Castle D, Mandell JW, Lee KS, Harris TH, Kipnis J. Structural and functional features of central nervous system lymphatic vessels. Nature 2015 July 16;523(7560):337–41.

13. "The 'Omics' Revolution: The Gut Microbiome," Institute for Functional Medicine video: https://vimeo.com/118612677?utm_source =AIC+Email+%233&utm_campaign=Aic+email+3+nonregistered& utm_medium=email.

14. Lyte M. Microbial endocrinology in the microbiome-gut-brain axis: How bacterial production and utilization of neurochemicals influence behavior. *PLoS Pathog.* 2013;9(11).

15. Alcock J, Maley CC, Aktipis CA. Is eating behavior manipulated by the gastrointestinal microbiota? Evolutionary pressures and potential mechanisms. *Bioessays.* 2014 Oct;36(10) 940–9.

16. Bercik P, Denou E, Collins J, et al. The intestinal microbiota affect central levels of brain-derived neurotropic factor and behavior in mice. *Gastroenterology.* 2011 Aug;14(2):599–609.

17. Rapid and unexpected weight gain after fecal transplant, Science-Daily, February 4, 2015: http://www.sciencedaily.com/releases/2015/02/150204125810.htm.

18. Bredesen DE. Reversal of cognitive decline: a novel therapeutic program. *Aging (Albany NY).* 2014 Sep;6(9):707–17.

Stage One: Activate a Biochemical Shift

1. Agah S, Mehdi Taleb A, Moeini R, Girji N, Nikbakht H. Cumin extract for symptom control in patients with irritable bowel syndrome: a case series. *Middle East J Dig Dis.* 2013 Oct; 5(4):217–22.

2. Nair V, Singh S, Gupta YK. Evaluation of disease modifying activity of *Coriandrum sativum* in experimental models. *Indian J Med Res.* 2012;135;240–5.

3. Beliga MS, Dsouza JJ. Amla (*Emblica officinalis* Gaertn.), a wonder berry in the treatment and prevention of cancer. *Eur J Cancer Prev.* 2011 May;20(3):225–39; Jose JK, Kuttan G, Kuttan R. Antitumour activity of *Emblica officinalis. J Ethnopharmacol.* 2001 May;75(2–3);65–69.

4. Akhtar MS, Ramzan A, Ali A, Ahmad M. Effect of Amla fruit (*Emblica officinalis* Gaertn.) on blood glucose and lipid profile of normal subjects and type 2 diabetic patients. *Int J Food Sci Nutr.* 2001 Sep;62(6):609–16.

5. Maruthappan V, Sakthi Shree K. Hypolipidemic activity of haritaki (*Terminalia chebula*) in atherogenic diet induced hyperlipidemic rats. *J Adv Pharm Technol Res*. 2010 Apr–June;1(2):229–35.

6. Babita Y, Sandhya Rani K, Sulochana B, Mamta S. A perspective study of haritaki. *Int J Res Ayurveda Pharm*. 2011;2(5):1466–70.

Stage Two: Crush Cravings (No Willpower Required)

1. Andallu B, Radhika B. Hypoglycemic, diuretic and hypocholesterolemic effect of Winter Cherry (*Withania somnifera*, Dunal) root. *Indian J Exp Biol*. 2000;38:607–9.

2. Mishra LC, Singh BB, Dagenais S. Scientific basis for the therapeutic use of *Withania somnifera* (ashwaganda): a review. *Altern Med Rev*. 2000 Aug;5(4):334–46.

3. Bhattacharya SK, Muruganandam AV. Adaptogenic activity of *Withania somnifera*: an experimental study using a rat model of chronic stress. *Pharmacol Biochem Be*. 2003;75(3):547–55.

4. Jain S, Shukla SD, Sharma K, Bhatnagar M. Neuroprotective effects of *Withania somnifera* Dunn. in hippocampal sub-regions of female albino rat. *Phytother Res*. 2001 Sep;15(6):544–8.

5. Roodenrys S, Booth D, Bulzomi S, Phipps A, Micallef C, Smoker J. Chronic effects of Brahmi (*Bacopa monnieri*) on human memory. *Neuropsychopharmacol*. 2002 Aug;27(2):279–81.

6. Rennard BO, Ertl RF, Gossman GL, Robbins RA, Rennard SI. Chicken soup inhibits neutrophil chemotaxis *in vitro*. *Chest*. 2000 Oct;118(4):1150–7.

7. Daniel KT. Why broth is beautiful: essential roles for proline, glycine, and gelatin. Weston A. Price Foundation post: http://www.westona price.org/health-topics/why-broth-is-beautiful-essential-roles-for -proline-glycine-and-gelatin/ (this article contains extensive relevant references).

Stage Three: Ignite Energy and Fat

1. Den R. Therapeutic effects of guggul and its constituent guggulsterone: cardiovascular benefits. *Cardiovasc Drug Rev*. 2007 Winter;25(4):375–90.

2. Shields KM, Moranville MP. Guggul for hypocholesterolemia. *Am J Health-Syst Ph*. 2005;62(10):1012–4.

3. Ernst E, Pittler MH. Efficacy of ginger for nausea and vomiting: a systematic review of randomized clinical trials. *Brit J Anaesth*. 2000;84(3):367–71.

4. Zick SM, Turgeon DK, Vareed SK, et al. Phase II study of the

effects of ginger root extract on eicosanoids in colon mucosa in people at normal risk for colorectal cancer. *Cancer Prev Res (Phila).* 2011;4(11):1929–37.

5.   Zick SM, Djuric Z, Ruffin MT, et al. Pharmacokinetics of 6-, 8-, 10-gingerols and 6-shagaol and conjugate metabolites in healthy human subjects. *Cancer Epidemiol Biomarkers Prev.* 2008 Aug;17(8):1930–6.

6.   Srinivasan M. Effect of curcumin on blood sugar as seen in a diabetic subject. *Indian J Med Sci.* 1972;26(4):269–70.

7.   Ramadan G, El-Menshawy O. Protective effects of ginger-turmeric rhizomes mixtures on joint inflammation, atherogenesis, kidney dysfunction and other complications in a rat model of human rheumatoid arthritis. *Int J Rheum Dis.* 2013 Apr;16(2):219–29.

8.   Srivastava KC, Bordia A, Verma SK. Curcumin, a major component of food spice turmeric (Curcuma longa) inhibits aggregation and alters eicosanoid metabolism in human blood platelets. *Prostaglandins Leuk of Essent Fatty Acids.* 1995;52(4):223–7.

9.   Oetari S, Sudibyo M, Commandeur JNM, Samhoedi R, Vermeulen NPE. Effects of curcumin on cytochrome P450 and glutathione S-transferase activities in rat liver. *Biochem Pharmacol.* 1996;51(1):39–45.

10. Bush JA, Cheung KJ Jr, Li G. Curcumin induces apoptosis in human melanoma cells through a Fas receptor/caspase-8 pathway independent of p53. *Exp Cell Res.* 2001 Dec 10;271(2):305–14.

11. Su CC, Lin JG, Li TM, et al. Curcumin-induced apoptosis of human colon cancer colo 205 cells through the production of ROS, Ca2+ and the activation of caspase-3. *Anticancer Res.* 2006 Nov–Dec;26(6B):4379–89.

12. Baum L, Ng A. Curcumin interaction with copper and iron suggests one possible mechanism of action in Alzheimer's disease animal models. *J Alzheimers Dis.* 2004 Aug;6(4):367–77.

Stage Four: Biohack Your Lifestyle Habits

1.   Shi S, Ansari T, McGuinness OP, Wasserman DH, Johnson CH. Circadian disruption leads to insulin resistance and obesity. *Curr Biol.* 2013;23(5):372–81.

2.   Kahleova H, Belinova L, Malinska H, et al. Eating two larger meals a day (breakfast and lunch) is more effective than six smaller meals in a reduced-energy regimen for patients with type 2 diabetes: a randomized crossover study. *Diabetologia.* 2015;58(1):205.

3.   Miglio C, Chiavaro E, Visconti A, Fogliano V, Pellegrin N. Effects of different cooking methods on nutritional and physiochemical char-

acteristics of selected vegetables. *J Agr Food Chem.* 2008;56(1):139–47.

4. Sudsuang R, Chentanez V, Velluvan K. Effect of Buddhist meditation on serum cortisol and total protein levels, blood pressure, pulse rate, lung volume, and reaction time. *Physiol Behav.* 1991;50(3):543–8.

5. Davidson RJ, Kabat-Zinn J, Schumacher J, et al. Alterations in brain and immune function produced by mindfulness meditation. *Psychosom Med.* 2003;65(4):564–70.

6. Morone N, Greco C, Weiner D. Mindfulness meditation for the treatment of chronic low back pain in older adults: a randomized controlled pilot study. *Pain.* 2008;134(3):310–9.

7. Shannahoff-Khalsa D. Complementary healthcare practices. Stress management for gastrointestinal disorders: the use of kundalini yoga meditation techniques. *Gastroenterol Nurs.* 2002 May–Jun;25(3):126–9.

8. Gaylord SA, Palsson OS, Garland EL, et al. Mindfulness training reduces the severity of irritable bowel syndrome in women: results of a randomized controlled study. *Am J Gastroenterol.* 2011;106:1678–88.

9. Tang YY, Ma Y, Wang J, et al. Short-term meditation training improves attention and self-regulation. *P Natl Acad Sci USA.* 2007;104(43):17152–6.

10. Kabat-Zinn J, Massion AO, Kristeller J, et al. Effectiveness of a meditation-based stress reduction program in the treatment of anxiety disorders. *Am J Psychiatry.* 1992 Jul;149(7):936–43.

11. Zylowska L, Ackerman DL, Yang MH, et al. Mindfulness meditation training in adults and adolescents with ADHD: a feasibility study. *J Atten Disord.* 2008 May;11(6):737–46.

12. Simpson TL, Kaysen D, Bowen S, et al. PTSD symptoms, substance use, and vipassana meditation among incarcerated individuals. *J Trauma Stress.* 2007;20(3):239–49.

13. Taheri S, Lin L, Austin D, Young T, Mignot E. Short sleep duration is associated with reduced leptin, elevated ghrelin, and increased body mass index. *PLoS Medicine.* 2004;e62. Epub: http://www.ncbi.nlm.nih.gov/pubmed/15602591.

Chapter 8: Ancient Food Knowledge for the Modern World

1. Akhtar MS, Ramzan A, Ali A, Ahmad M. Effect of Amla fruit (*Emblica officinalis* Gaertn.) on blood glucose and lipid profile of normal subjects and type 2 diabetic patients. *Int J Food Sci Nutr.* 2001 Sep;62(6):609–16.

2. Hishikawa N, Takahashi Y, Amakusa Y, et al. Effects of turmeric on Alzheimer's disease with behavioral and psychological symptoms of dementia. *AYU: International Quarterly Journal of Research in Ayurveda.* 2012;33(4):499–504.

3. Some statistics show death rates from Alzheimer's to be much lower in India. For example: Alzheimer's/dementia death rates per 100,000, age-standardized per country, from World Health Rankings: http://www.worldlifeexpectancy.com/cause-of-death/alzheimers -dementia/by-country/. Some studies show that Alzheimer's incidence is only marginally lower than in Western regions such as the United States and Europe. For example, see Mathuranath PS, George A, Ranijth N, et al. Incidence of Alzheimer's disease in India: a 10 years follow-up study. *Neurol India.* 2012;60(6):625–30.

4. Brown RJ, DeBanate MA, Rother KI. Artificial sweeteners: a systematic review of metabolic effects in youth. *Int J Pediatr Obes.* 2010;5(4):305–12.

5. Suez J, Korem T, Zeevi D, et al. Artificial sweeteners induce glucose intolerance by altering the gut microbiota. *Nature.* 2014;514:181–186.

6. Yang Q. Gain weight by "going diet?" Artificial sweeteners and the neurobiology of sugar cravings. *Yale J Biol Med.* 2010;83(2):101–8.

7. Annapoorani A, Anilakumar KR, Khanum F, Murthy NA, Bawa AS. Studies on the physiochemical characteristics of heated honey, honey mixed with *ghee* and their food consumption pattern by rats. *AYU: International Quarterly Journal of Research in Ayurveda.* 2010;31(2): 141–6.

8. Meydani SN, Ha WK. Immunologic effects of yogurt. *Am J Clin Nutr.* 2000;71(4):861–72. See also Saavedra JM, Tschernia A. Human studies with probiotics and prebiotics: clinical implications. *Brit J Nutr.* 2002;87(2 Suppl):241–6.

9. Jacques PF, Wang H. Yogurt and weight management. *Am J Clin Nutr.* 2014;99(5 Suppl):1229–34.

10. Snowdon DA, Phillips RL, Fraser GE. Meat consumption and fatal ischemic heart disease. *Prev Med.* 1984;13(5):490–500.

11. Micha R, Wallace SK, Mozaffarian D. Red and processed meat consumption and risk of incident coronary heart disease, stroke, and diabetes: a systematic review and meta-analysis. *Circulation.* 2010;121(21):2271–83.

12. Pan A, Sun Q, Bernstein AM, Manson JE, Willett WC, Hu FB. Changes in red meat consumption and subsequent risk of type 2 diabetes mellitus: three cohorts of US men and women. *JAMA Intern Med.* 2013;173(14):1328–35.

13. Craig WJ. Health effects of vegan diets. *Am J Clin Nutr.* 2009;89(5):1627S–33S.
14. Key TJ, Fraser GE, Thorogood M, et al. Mortality in vegetarians and nonvegetarians: detailed findings from a collaborative analysis of 5 prospective studies. *Am J Clin Nutr.* 1999;70(3):516–24.
15. Regional Office for Asia and the Pacific, *Guidelines for Humane Handling, Transport, and Slaughter of Livestock*, Chapter 2: "Effects of Stress and Injury on Meat and By-product Quality": http://www.fao .org/docrep/003/x6909e/x6909e04.htm.
16. Korneliussen I. Is meat from stressed animals unhealthy? Published online by ScienceNordic: http://sciencenordic.com/meat-stressed -animals-unhealthy.
17. Daley CA, Abbott A, Doyle P, Nader GA, Larson S. A review of fatty acid profiles and antioxidant content in grass-fed and grain-fed beef. *Nutr J.* 2010 Mar 10;9:10.
18. Sharma H, Zhang X, Dwivedi C. The effect of *ghee* (clarified butter) on serum lipid levels and microsomal lipid peroxidation. *AYU: International Quarterly Journal of Research in Ayurveda.* 2010;31(2):134–40.

Chapter 10: More Ayurvedic Wisdom for the Rest of Your Life

1. Li X, Kolltveit KM, Tronstad L, Olsen I. Systemic diseases caused by oral infection. *Clin Microbiol Rev.* 2000;13(4):547–58.
2. Joshipura KJ, Rimm EB, Douglass CW, Trichopoulos D, Ascherio A, Willett WC. Poor oral health and coronary heart disease. *J Dent Res.* 1996 Sep;75(9):1631–6.
3. Singh A, Purohit B. Tooth brushing, oil pulling, and tissue regeneration: a review of holistic approaches to oral health. *J Ayurveda Integr Med.* 2011;2(2):64–8.
4. Pedrazzi V, Sato S, de Mattos G, Lara EH, Panzeri H. Tongue-cleaning methods: a comparative clinical trial employing a toothbrush and a tongue scraper. *J Periodontol.* 2004;75(7):1009–12.
5. Andrade AM, Greene GW, Melanson KJ. Eating slowly led to decreases in energy intake within meals in healthy women. *J Am Diet Assoc.* 2008;108(7):1186–91.
6. George DF, Bilek MM, McKenzie DR. Microwaves cause a significantly higher degree of unfolding than conventional thermal stress for protein solutions heated to the same maximum temperature. *Bioelectromagnetics.* 2008;29(4):324–30.
7. Conboy LA, Edshteyn I, Garivaltis H. Ayurveda and panchakarma: measuring the effects of a holistic health intervention. *Scientific World Journal.* 2009;9:272–80.

8. Sharma HM, Nidich SI, Sands D, Smith DE. Improvement in cardio-vascular risk factors through panchakarma purification procedures. *J Res Educ Indian Med.* 1993;12(4):3–13.
9. Herron RE, Fagan JB. Lipophil-mediated reduction of toxicants in humans: an evaluation of an Ayurvedic detoxification procedure. *Altern Ther Health Med.* 2002 Sep–Oct;8(5):40–51.

BIBLIOGRAPHY

Agah S, Mehdi Taleb A, Moeini R, Girji N, Nikbakht H. Cumin extract for symptom control in patients with irritable bowel syndrome: a case series. *Middle East J Dig Dis.* 2013 Oct;5(4):217–22.

Agriculture Fact Book, Chapter 2, "Profiling Food Consumption in America": http://www.usda.gov/factbook/chapter2.pdf.

Akhtar MS, Ramzan A, Ali A, Ahmad M. Effect of Amla fruit (*Emblica officinalis* Gaertn.) on blood glucose and lipid profile of normal subjects and type 2 diabetic patients. *Int J Food Sci Nutr.* 2001 Sep;62(6):609–16.

Alcock J, Maley CC, Aktipis CA. Is eating behavior manipulated by the gastrointestinal microbiota? Evolutionary pressures and potential mechanisms. *Bioessays.* 2014;36(10):940–9.

Andallu B, Radhika B. Hypoglycemic, diuretic and hypocholesterolemic effect of Winter Cherry (*Withania somnifera*, Dunal) root. *Indian J Exp Biol.* 2000;38:607–9.

Andrade AM, Greene GW, Melanson KJ. Eating slowly led to decreases in energy intake within meals in healthy women. *J Am Diet Assoc.* 2008;108(7):1186–91.

Annapoorani A, Anilakumar KR, Khanum F, Murthy NA, Bawa AS. Studies on the physiochemical characteristics of heated honey, honey mixed with *ghee* and their food consumption pattern by rats. *AYU: International Quarterly Journal of Research in Ayurveda.* 2010;31(2): 141–6.

Autoimmune statistics from the American Autoimmune Related Diseases Association, Inc.: http://www.aarda.org/autoimmune-information/autoimmune-statistics/.

Babita Y, Sandhya Rani K, Sulochana B, Mamta S. A perspective study of haritaki. *Int J Res Ayurveda Pharm.* 2011;2(5):1466–70.

"Background on Chemicals and Waste," United Nations Environment Programme: http://www.unep.org/chemicalsandwaste/Introduction/BackgroundonChemicalsandWaste/tabid/1059847/Default.aspx.

Barry D, Clarke M, Petry N. Obesity and its relationship to addictions: is overeating a form of addictive behavior? *Am J Addict.* 2009:18(6): 439–51.

Baum L, Ng A. Curcumin interaction with copper and iron suggests one possible mechanism of action in Alzheimer's disease animal models. *J Alzheimers Dis.* 2004 Aug;6(4):367–77.

Beliga MS, Dsouza JJ. Amla (*Emblica officinalis* Gaertn.), a wonder berry in the treatment and prevention of cancer. *Eur J Cancer Prev.* 2011 May;20(3):225–39.

Bercik P, Denou E, Collins J, et al. The intestinal microbiota affect central levels of brain-derived neurotropic factor and behavior in mice. *Gastroenterology.* 2011 Aug;14(2):599–609.

Bhattacharya SK, Muruganandam AV. Adaptogenic activity of *Withania somnifera*: an experimental study using a rat model of chronic stress. *Pharmacol Biochem Be.* 2003;75(3):547–55.

"Body Burden: The Pollution in Newborns," The Environmental Working Group, July 14, 2005: http://www.ewg.org/research/body-burden-pollution-newborns.

Braak H, Rub U, Gai WP, Del Tredici K. Idiopathic Parkinson's disease: possible routes by which vulnerable neuronal types may be subject to neuroinvasion by an unknown pathogen. *J Neural Transm.* 2003;110(5):517–36.

Bredesen DE. Reversal of cognitive decline: a novel therapeutic program. *Aging (Albany NY).* 2014 Sep;6(9):707–17.

Brown RJ, DeBanate MA, Rother KI. Artificial sweeteners: a systematic review of metabolic effects in youth. *Int J Pediatr Obes.* 2010;5(4): 305–12.

Bush JA, Cheung KJ Jr, Li G. Curcumin induces apoptosis in human melanoma cells through a Fas receptor/caspase-8 pathway independent of p53. *Exp Cell Res.* 2001 Dec 10;271(2):305–14.

Camilleri M. Serotonin in the gastrointestinal tract. *Curr Opin Endocrinol Diabetes Obes.* 2009;16(1):53–9.

Ch'ng CL, Jones MK, Kingham JGC. Celiac disease and autoimmune thyroid disease. *Clin Med Res.* 2007;5(3):184–92.

Cohen J. Faster environmental testing for new synthetic chemicals and materials. *UC Santa Barbara Current*, Science + Technology section, April 10, 2014: http://www.news.ucsb.edu/2014/014070/faster-environmental-testing-new-synthetic-chemicals-and-materials.

Collins SM, Surette M, Bercik P. The interplay between the intestinal microbiota and the brain. *Nat Rev Microbiol.* 2012 Nov;10(11):735–42.

Conboy LA, Edshteyn I, Garivaltis H. Ayurveda and panchakarma: measuring the effects of a holistic health intervention. *Scientific World Journal.* 2009;9:272–80.

Corcoran C, Thomas P, O'Keane V. Vagus nerve stimulation in chronic treatment-resistant depression. *Brit J Psychiat.* 2006;189:282–3.

Craig WJ. Health effects of vegan diets. *Am J Clin Nutr.* 2009;89(5):1627S–33S.

Creamer B, Shorter RG, Bamforth J. The turnover and shedding of epithelia cells, Part I: The turnover in the gastro-intestinal tract. *Gut.* 1961:2,110.

Cyrex Laboratories, http://www.cyrexlabs.com.

Daley CA, Abbott A, Doyle P, Nader GA, Larson S. A review of fatty acid profiles and antioxidant content in grass-fed and grain-fed beef. *Nutr J.* 2010 Mar 10;9:10.

Daniel KT. Why broth is beautiful: essential roles for proline, glycine, and gelatin. Weston A. Price Foundation post: http://www.westonaprice.org/health-topics/why-broth-is-beautiful-essential-roles-for-proline-glycine-and-gelatin/ (this article contains extensive relevant references).

Davidson RJ, Kabat-Zinn J, Schumacher J, et al. Alterations in brain and immune function produced by mindfulness meditation. *Psychosom Med.* 2003;65(4):564–70.

Del Tredici K, Rub U, De Vos R, Bohl J, Braak H. Where does Parkinson's disease pathology begin in the brain? *J Neuropath Exp Neur.* 2002 May:61(5):413–26.

Den R. Therapeutic effects of guggul and its constituent guggulsterone: cardiovascular benefits. *Cardiovasc Drug Rev.* 2007 Winter;25(4):375–90.

Dutta G, Zhang P, Liu B. The lipopolysaccharide Parkinson's disease animal model: mechanistic studies and drug recovery. *Fundam Clin Pharmacol.* 2008 Oct;22(5):453–64.

Ernst E, Pittler MH. Efficacy of ginger for nausea and vomiting: a systematic review of randomized clinical trials. *Brit J Anaesth.* 2000;84(3): 367–71.

Fasano A. Zonulin and its regulation of intestinal barrier function: the biological door to inflammation, autoimmunity, and cancer. *Physiol Rev.* 2011 Jan;91(1):151–75.

Fasano A, Shea-Donohue T. Mechanisms of disease: the role of intestinal barrier function in the pathogenesis of gastrointestinal autoimmune diseases. *Nat Clin Pract Gastroenterol Hepatol.* 2005:2,416–22.

Gaylord SA, Palsson OS, Garland EL, et al. Mindfulness training reduces the severity of irritable bowel syndrome in women: results of a randomized controlled study. *Am J Gastroenterol.* 2011;106:1678–88.

George DF, Bilek MM, McKenzie DR. Microwaves cause a significantly higher degree of unfolding than conventional thermal stress for protein solutions heated to the same maximum temperature. *Bioelectromagnetics.* 2008;29(4):324–30.

Herron RE, Fagan JB. Lipophil-mediated reduction of toxicants in humans: an evaluation of an Ayurvedic detoxification procedure. *Altern Ther Health Med.* 2002 Sep–Oct;8(5):40–51.

Hishikawa N, Takahashi Y, Amakusa Y, et al. Effects of turmeric on Alzheimer's disease with behavioral and psychological symptoms of dementia. *AYU: International Quarterly Journal of Research in Ayurveda.* 2012;33(4):499–504.

Holmqvist S, Chutna O, Bousset L, et al. Direct evidence of Parkinson pathology spread from the gastrointestinal tract to the brain in rats. *Acta Neuropathol.* 2014;128(6):805–20.

Jacques PF, Wang H. Yogurt and weight management. *Am J Clin Nutr.* 2014;99(5 Suppl):1229–34.

Jain S, Shukla SD, Sharma K, Bhatnagar M. Neuroprotective effects of *Withania somnifera* Dunn. in hippocampal sub-regions of female albino rat. *Phytother Res.* 2001 Sep;15(6):544–8.

Johnson RJ, Segal MS, Sautin Y, et al. Potential role of sugar (fructose) in the epidemic of hypertension, obesity, and the metabolic syndrome, diabetes, kidney disease, and cardiovascular disease. *Am J Clin Nutr.* 2007 Oct;86(4):899–906.

Jose JK, Kuttan G, Kuttan R. Antitumour activity of *Emblica officinalis*. *J Ethnopharmacol.* 2001 May;75(2–3);65–69.

Joshipura KJ, Rimm EB, Douglass CW, Trichopoulos D, Ascherio A, Willett WC. Poor oral health and coronary heart disease. *J Dent Res.* 1996 Sep;75(9):1631–6.

Kabat-Zinn J, Massion AO, Kristeller J, et al. Effectiveness of a meditation-based stress reduction program in the treatment of anxiety disorders. *Am J Psychiatry.* 1992 Jul;149(7):936–43.

Kahleova H, Belinova L, Malinska H, et al. Eating two larger meals a day (breakfast and lunch) is more effective than six smaller meals in a reduced-energy regimen for patients with type 2 diabetes: a randomized crossover study. *Diabetologia.* 2015;58(1):205.

Key TJ, Fraser GE, Thorogood M, et al. Mortality in vegetarians and non-vegetarians: detailed findings from a collaborative analysis of 5 prospective studies. *Am J Clin Nutr.* 1999;70(3):516–24.

Korneliussen I. Is meat from stressed animals unhealthy? Published online by ScienceNordic: http://sciencenordic.com/meat-stressed-animals-unhealthy.

Li X, Kolltveit KM, Tronstad L, Olsen I. Systemic diseases caused by oral infection. *Clin Microbiol Rev.* 2000;13(4):547–58.

Lim JS, Lee DH, Park JY, Jin SH, Jacobs DR Jr. A strong interaction between serum gamma-glutamyltransferase and obesity on the risk of prevalent type 2 diabetes: results from the Third National Health and Nutrition Examination Survey. *Clin Chem.* 2007;53(6):1092–109.

Louveau A, Smirnov I, Keyes TJ, Eccles JD, Rouhani SJ, Peske JD, Derecki NC, Castle D, Mandell JW, Lee KS, Harris TH, Kipnis J. Structural and functional features of central nervous system lymphatic vessels. *Nature* 2015 July 16;523(7560):337–41.

Lyte M. Microbial endocrinology in the microbiome-gut-brain axis: How bacterial production and utilization of neurochemicals influence behavior. *PLoS Pathog.* 2013;9(11).

Malik VS, Schulze MB, Hu FB. Intake of sugar-sweetened beverages and weight gain: a systematic review. *Am J Clin Nutr.* 2006 Aug;84(2):274–88.

Maruthappan V, Sakthi Shree K. Hypolipidemic activity of haritaki (*Terminalia chebula*) in atherogenic diet induced hyperlipidemic rats. *J Adv Pharm Technol Res.* 2010 Apr–June;1(2):229–35.

Meydani SN, Ha WK. Immunologic effects of yogurt. *Am J Clin Nutr.* 2000;71(4):861–72. See also Saavedra JM, Tschernia A. Human studies with probiotics and prebiotics: clinical implications. *Brit J Nutr.* 2002;87(2 Suppl):241–6.

Micha R, Wallace SK, Mozaffarian D. Red and processed meat consumption and risk of incident coronary heart disease, stroke, and diabetes: a systematic review and meta-analysis. *Circulation.* 2010;121(21):2271–83.

Miglio C, Chiavaro E, Visconti A, Fogliano V, Pellegrin N. Effects of different cooking methods on nutritional and physiochemical characteristics of selected vegetables. *J Agr Food Chem.* 2008;56(1):139–47.

Mishra LC, Singh BB, Dagenais S. Scientific basis for the therapeutic use of *Withania somnifera* (ashwaganda): a review. *Altern Med Rev.* 2000 Aug;5(4):334–46.

Moreira MA, Andre LC, Cardeal ZL. Analysis of plasticizer migration to meat roasted in plastic bags by SPME-GC/MS. *Food Chem.* 2015;178:195–200.

Morone N, Greco C, Weiner D. Mindfulness meditation for the treatment of chronic low back pain in older adults: a randomized controlled pilot study. *Pain.* 2008;134(3):310–9.

Nair V, Singh S, Gupta YK. Evaluation of disease modifying activity of *Coriandrum sativum* in experimental models. *Indian J Med Res.* 2012;135;240–5.

Oetari S, Sudibyo M, Commandeur JNM, Samhoedi R, Vermeulen NPE. Effects of curcumin on cytochrome P450 and glutathione S-transferase activities in rat liver. *Biochem Pharmacol.* 1996;51(1):39–45.

Pan A, Sun Q, Bernstein AM, Manson JE, Willett WC, Hu FB. Changes in red meat consumption and subsequent risk of type 2 diabetes mellitus: three cohorts of US men and women. *JAMA Intern Med.* 2013;173(14):1328–35.

Pedrazzi V, Sato S, de Mattos G, Lara EH, Panzeri H. Tongue-cleaning methods: a comparative clinical trial employing a toothbrush and a tongue scraper. *J Periodontol.* 2004;75(7):1009–12.

Pereira MA, Kartashov Al, Ebbeling CB, et al. Fast-food habits, weight gain, and insulin resistance (the CARDIA study): 15-year prospective analysis. *Lancet.* 2005;366(9464):1030.

Prat A, Biernacki K, Wosik K, Antel JP. Glial influence on the human blood-brain barrier. *Glia.* 2001;36(2):145–55.

Ramadan G, El-Menshawy O. Protective effects of ginger-turmeric rhizomes mixtures on joint inflammation, atherogenesis, kidney dysfunction and other complications in a rat model of human rheumatoid arthritis. *Int J Rheum Dis.* 2013 Apr;16(2):219–29.

Rapid and unexpected weight gain after fecal transplant, *ScienceDaily,* February 4, 2015: http://www.sciencedaily.com/releases/2015/02/150204125810.htm.

Regional Office for Asia and the Pacific, *Guidelines for Humane Handling, Transport, and Slaughter of Livestock,* Chapter 2: "Effects of Stress and Injury on Meat and By-product Quality": http://www.fao.org/docrep/003/x6909e/x6909e04.htm.

Rennard BO, Ertl RF, Gossman GL, Robbins RA, Rennard SI. Chicken soup inhibits neutrophil chemotaxis *in vitro. Chest.* 2000 Oct;118(4):1150–7.

Roodenrys S, Booth D, Bulzomi S, Phipps A, Micallef C, Smoker J. Chronic effects of Brahmi (*Bacopa monnieri*) on human memory. *Neuropsychopharmacol.* 2002 Aug;27(2):279–81.

Ruhl A. Glial cells in the gut. *Neurogastroent Motil.* 2005;17(6):777–90.

Savidge TC, Newman P, Pothoulakis C, et al. Enteric glia regulate intestinal barrier function and inflammation via release of S-nitrosoglutathione. *Gastroenterology.* 2007 Apr;132(4):1344–58.

Shannahoff-Khalsa D. Complementary healthcare practices. Stress management for gastrointestinal disorders: the use of kundalini yoga meditation techniques. *Gastroenterol Nurs.* 2002 May–Jun;25(3):126–9.

Sharma H, Zhang X, Dwivedi C. The effect of *ghee* (clarified butter) on serum lipid levels and microsomal lipid peroxidation. *AYU: International Quarterly Journal of Research in Ayurveda.* 2010;31(2):134–40.

Sharma HM, Nidich SI, Sands D, Smith DE. Improvement in cardiovascular risk factors through panchakarma purification procedures. *J Res Educ Indian Med.* 1993;12(4):3–13.

Shi S, Ansari T, McGuinness OP, Wasserman DH, Johnson CH. Circadian disruption leads to insulin resistance and obesity. *Curr Biol.* 2013;23(5):372–81.

Shields KM, Moranville MP. Guggul for hypocholesterolemia. *Am J Health-Syst Ph.* 2005;62(10):1012–4.

Simpson TL, Kaysen D, Bowen S, et al. PTSD symptoms, substance use, and vipassana meditation among incarcerated individuals. *J Trauma Stress.* 2007;20(3):239–49.

Singh A, Purohit B. Tooth brushing, oil pulling, and tissue regeneration: a review of holistic approaches to oral health. *J Ayurveda Integr Med.* 2011;2(2):64–8.

Snowdon DA, Phillips RL, Fraser GE. Meat consumption and fatal ischemic heart disease. *Prev Med.* 1984;13(5):490–500.

Some statistics show death rates from Alzheimer's to be much lower in India. For example: Alzheimer's/dementia death rates per 100,000, age-standardized per country, from World Health Rankings: http://www .worldlifeexpectancy.com/cause-of-death/alzheimers-dementia/by -country/. Some studies show that Alzheimer's incidence is only marginally lower than in Western regions such as the United States and Europe. For example, see Mathuranath PS, George A, Ranijth N, et al. Incidence of Alzheimer's disease in India: a 10 years follow-up study. *Neurol India.* 2012;60(6):625–30.

Srinivasan M. Effect of curcumin on blood sugar as seen in a diabetic subject. *Indian J Med Sci.* 1972;26(4):269–70.

Srivastava KC, Bordia A, Verma SK. Curcumin, a major component of food spice turmeric (*Curcuma longa*) inhibits aggregation and alters eicosanoid metabolism in human blood platelets. *Prostaglandins Leuk of Essent Fatty Acids.* 1995;52(4):223–7.

Su CC, Lin JG, Li TM, et al. Curcumin-induced apoptosis of human colon cancer colo 205 cells through the production of ROS, Ca2+ and the activation of caspase-3. *Anticancer Res.* 2006 Nov–Dec;26(6B):4379–89.

Sudsuang R, Chentanez V, Velluvan K. Effect of Buddhist meditation on serum cortisol and total protein levels, blood pressure, pulse rate, lung volume, and reaction time. *Physiol Behav.* 1991;50(3):543–8.

Suez J, Korem T, Zeevi D, et al. Artificial sweeteners induce glucose intolerance by altering the gut microbiota. *Nature: International Weekly Journal of Science.* 2014;514:181–6.

Taheri S, Lin L, Austin D, Young T, Mignot E. Short sleep duration is associated with reduced leptin, elevated ghrelin, and increased body mass index. *PLoS Medicine.* 2004;e62. Epub: http://www.ncbi.nlm .nih.gov/pubmed/15602591.

Tang YY, Ma Y, Wang J, et al. Short-term meditation training improves attention and self-regulation. *P Natl Acad Sci USA.* 2007;104(43): 17152–6.

"The 'Omics' Revolution: The Gut Microbiome," Institute for Functional Medicine video: https://vimeo.com/118612677?utm_source=AIC

+Email+%233&utm_campaign=Aic+email+3+nonregistered&utm _medium=email.

"The Sensitive Gut," a Harvard Medical School Special Health Report prepared in consultation with Lawrence S. Friedman, M.D., 2012.

Van Oudenhove L, McKie S, Lassman D, et al. Fatty acid-induced gutbrain signaling attenuates neural and behavioral effects of sad emotion in humans. *J Clin Invest.* 2011;121(8):3094–9.

Visser J, Rozing J, Sapone A, Lammers K, Fasano A. Tight junctions, intestinal permeability, and autoimmunity celiac disease and type 1 diabetes paradigms. *Ann N Y Acad Sci.* 2009;1165:195–205.

WebMD article discussing the medical status of leaky gut syndrome: http:// www.webmd.com/digestive-disorders/features/leaky-gut-syndrome.

Worldometers, which tracks toxic chemical release by industry on a real-time counter: http://www.worldometers.info/view/toxchem/.

Yang Q. Gain weight by "going diet?" Artificial sweeteners and the neurobiology of sugar cravings. *Yale J Biol Med.* 2010;83(2):101–8.

Yang Q, Zhang Z, Flanders WD, Merritt R, Hu FB. Added sugar intake and cardiovascular diseases mortality among US adults. *JAMA Intern Med.* 2014;174(4):516–24.

Zick SM, Djuric Z, Ruffin MT, et al. Pharmacokinetics of 6-, 8-, 10-gingerols and 6-shagaol and conjugate metabolites in healthy human subjects. *Cancer Epidemiol Biomarkers Prev.* 2008 Aug;17(8):1930–6.

Zick SM, Turgeon DK, Vareed SK, et al. Phase II study of the effects of ginger root extract on eicosanoids in colon mucosa in people at normal risk for colorectal cancer. *Cancer Prev Res (Phila).* 2011;4(11):1929–37.

Zylowska L, Ackerman DL, Yang MH, et al. Mindfulness meditation training in adults and adolescents with ADHD: a feasibility study. *J Atten Disord.* 2008 May;11(6):737–46.

RESOURCES

For more information on what I do and to find a source for all the supplements mentioned in the book, as well as other products including raw silk gloves for lymphatic massage, see my website: www.drkulreetchaudhary .com.

You can also find all the supplements recommended in this book on the website for VPK by Maharishi Ayurveda (MAPI), at www.myvpk.com /theprime. While you can certainly use other brands, this is the brand that produces the supplements I helped formulate. They are the ones I use and recommend.

To find a Transcendental Meditation Teacher, visit www.tm.org.

To find an Ayurvedic practitioner near you, a great source is the National Ayurvedic Medical Association at www.ayurvedanama.org.

To learn more about endobiogeny, go to www.endobiogeny.com.

To learn more about functional medicine, visit www.functionalmedicine .org.

For a good source of bone broth, try out www.bonebroth.com.

ACKNOWLEDGMENTS

I'd like to thank my family: Joshua for his unwavering devotion; Sandeep for helping me create space in my life for creativity; Laura for her perpetual optimism about my ability to help others; Harleen for being the "cupcake" of the family; my mom for introducing me to Ayurveda and meditation; and Sathya and Suryani for bringing so much laughter into our lives.

I'd also like to thank my writer, Eve, who captured the tone of my heart and mind so effortlessly, and my agent, Alex, for igniting the idea of this book. Thanks to Heather, my editor, for being so ridiculously good at her job, and to my entire team at Penguin Random House for their enthusiasm and hard work. You've given me an extraordinary opportunity to help people.

Finally, I'd like to thank my CEO and dear friend, Steve, for believing we should build a healthcare company based on compassion, integrity, current research, and a genuine desire to heal people's lives.

INDEX

gluten, 51, 92, 93, 103, 111, 205–207, 217, 253
glycine, 149–150
glycogen, 82, 224
grains, 26, 196, 201–204, 209
grass-fed meat, 225
Graves' disease (hyperthyroidism), 93, 147
growth hormones, 220–221
guggul, 37, 85, 91, 94, 159, 160, 163–164, 169, 171, 174, 177, 178, 181, 188, 189
gums, 76, 257–258
gut bacteria (microbiome), 30, 33, 37, 72, 80, 90, 91, 98–99, 104, 106–110, 123
gut-blood-brain-barrier (GBBB), 102–104
Gut IQ Test, 117–120, 123, 134, 139, 168, 185, 217, 220, 254

habits (*see* Stage Four of The Prime)
halitosis, 257
haritaki berries, 36, 134, 135–136
Hashimoto's disease, 6, 93
headaches, 8–11, 14, 17, 34, 100, 138, 170
heart disease, 45, 51, 162
heartburn, 160, 164
heavy metals, 44, 94
hepatotoxin, 82
herbs (*see* specific herbs)
heroin, 48, 61
high-fructose corn syrup, 28, 45
Himalayan salt, 70, 220, 226
Hinduism, 12
homeostasis, 60, 61, 64, 73, 144
homogenization, 216
honey, 208, 211, 226
HPA axis, 60–61, 66, 71–73
hyperthyroidism (Graves' disease), 147
hypothalamus, 60

immune system, 86, 103
immunosuppressants, 92
indigestion, 78, 100, 131, 132, 189

Infectious Disease Society of America, 108
inflammation, 19, 20, 28–30, 33, 35, 40, 43, 74, 76, 91–93, 123, 132, 167, 203, 241, 263
insomnia, 110
Institute of Functional Medicine, 49, 106
insulin, 27, 83, 209
insulin resistance, 176
integrative medicine, 48–50
intermittent fasting, 265–266, 268
intolerances and sensitivities to food, 214–215
iron, 131
irritability, 160, 169, 170, 181
irritable bowel syndrome (IBS), 7, 99, 132, 180, 182

jaggery, 207, 208, 226
joint pain, 20, 170
Journal of the American Medical Association, 27
junk food, 19, 61, 64, 68, 144–145

kapha type, 229, 245–251
  fasting and, 267–268
  foods good for, 247–248
  foods to avoid, 248–249
  lifestyle for, 250–251
  sample meal plan, 250
  vegan diet and, 253
kidneys, 42, 125

lactase deficiency, 215
lactic acid, 224
lacto-ovo vegetarians, 223
large intestine (colon), 42, 80, 83, 106, 125, 133–135, 161, 169, 262
lassi, 150, 185–186, 190, 213, 216, 218–219, 221
  recipe for, 219–220
laxatives, 133
leaky gut syndrome, 90–93, 104, 109, 110, 215
legumes, 212

traditional Chinese medicine, 48
trans fats, 45
Transcendental Meditation (TM), 6, 182
trauma, 41, 43
tremors, 9
triphala, 11, 36, 91, 126, 133–137, 143, 161, 163, 171, 175, 185, 187
turbinado sugar, 226
turmeric, 4, 5, 91, 111, 166–167, 204, 216

ulcers, 78
unrefined cane sugar, 208
urinary problems, 16
urination, 125, 128
urine, odor of, 46

vagus nerve, 80, 97, 98, 101, 122, 263
vata type, 229, 235–240
    fasting and, 266–267
    foods good for, 237–238
    foods to avoid, 238–239
    lifestyle for, 239–240
    paleo diet and, 252
    sample meal plan, 239
Vedas, 12
vegans, 223, 238, 253

vegetable soup, 152
vegetables, raw, 38, 179–180
vegetarians, 150, 190, 201, 223
vitamin C, 180
vomiting, 122
VPK, 134, 222

Walmart, 31
water consumption, 21, 140
weight gain, 8, 9, 14, 18, 47–48, 91, 120, 210, 236, 240–241, 246–247
weight loss, 19–20, 23–31, 33–35, 74, 122–123, 184, 236
Western medicine, 4, 13, 16, 35, 41, 48–52, 112
wheat, 205–207
white blood cells, 102
whole food, 196, 199–201
Whole Foods, 157
whole grains, 197
willpower, 24–26, 31, 66–68, 70, 123, 141
withdrawal symptoms, 62, 63, 69

yogurt, 216, 218–220

zonulin, 92

ABOUT THE AUTHOR

Dr. Kulreet Chaudhary's combined expertise in both modern neurology and the ancient science of health known as Ayurveda has uniquely positioned her as an expert. She is passionate about raising awareness of the need for a paradigm shift in contemporary medicine that focuses on patient empowerment and a health-based (rather than disease-based) medical system. Dr. Chaudhary is a frequent guest on *The Dr. Oz Show,* where her teachings about Ayurvedic medicine have been applauded by a national audience.

Dr. Chaudhary was the director of Wellspring Health in Scripps Memorial Hospital for ten years and remains a pioneer in the field of integrative medicine. She has successfully developed a powerful system to manage chronic neurological disorders such as multiple sclerosis, Parkinson's disease, and migraine headaches by incorporating fundamental changes in diet, behavior, and stress, in addition to the standard allopathic approach to these issues. This program has been so successful that many patients now use it not just for neurological issues but also for a wider range of health concerns, including weight issues and chronic disease.

Dr. Chaudhary now serves as the chief medical officer for New Practices, Inc., where she is changing allopathic medical practices into healing centers using compassion-based health coaching, meditation, and integrative medicine to combat chronic diseases such as Alzheimer's disease, diabetes, obesity, coronary heart disease, depression, and more. She also oversees ongoing research in the management and reversal of chronic disease through lifestyle intervention. Dr. Chaudhary is creating a new model for healthcare that is based on teaching patients the principles of health and personal transformation in an environment of compassion, empowering them to live in a way that promotes maximum healing and vitality.

Dr. Kulreet Chaudhary is also a neuroscientist. She has participated in over twenty clinical research studies in the areas of multiple sclerosis, Alzheimer's disease, Parkinson's disease, ALS, and diabetic peripheral neuropathy. Her research includes groundbreaking work in stem cell therapies for diabetic peripheral neuropathy and drug development for the treatment of ALS.